Fertility and
Family Planning in a
Canadian Metropolis

Fertility and in

T. R. Balakrishnan
J. F. Kantner
J. D. Allingham

Family Planning a Canadian Metropolis

McGill–Queen's University Press
Montreal and London 1975

ISBN: 0 7735 0204 1
Legal Deposit Second Quarter 1975
Bibliothèque nationale du Québec
Design by Peter Maher
Printed in Canada by
The Bryant Press Limited

This book has been published with the help of a grant from the Social Science Research Council of Canada, using funds provided by the Canada Council.

Table of Contents

Tables

Table *Page*

Figures

Preface

This study stems from our interest in understanding the fertility behaviour of Canadian women. Our curiosity was aroused initially by the steady decline of the birth rate since the beginning of the sixties—a trend that was continuing unabated at the time the survey went into the field. This was the period when oral contraception was being rapidly adopted and when such basic issues as equality for women, liberalization of abortion laws, and attention of the family role structure were claiming public attention. Studies of fertility in the United States had shown that some of the long-standing relationships taken for granted in the past no longer held. Whether the findings from U.S. studies might be reasonably valid for the Canadian scene was itself a matter worth investigating. For these varied reasons then a study of fertility among Canadian women appeared to us to have high priority on the Canadian scientific agenda.

The accustomed mode of demographic investigation in Canada has been the analysis of secondary data provided by official statistical agencies. Useful as these have been they have not been able to probe the subject to any great depth. Not only do official statistics steer clear of the subject of contraception—knowledge of which is necessary to know the extent to which fertility behaviour reflects intention rather than chance—but they neglect also certain relevant dimensions of fertility such as the spacing of births, desired family size, and future birth expectations. Moreover, detailed field investigations can go much further in gathering information on the social and psychological context in which fertility and contraceptive behaviour occur. This study thus attempts to push beyond conventional analyses of demographic levels and trends into some of the underlying relationships.

Although large sums have occasionally been made available for social science research in Canada such as the amount spent for research by the B&B Commission, support for original investigation by university-based social scientists has been modest relative to amounts spent on other branches of science, or, more importantly, relative to the need for such research. Thus, though we recognized the need for a study that would be descriptive of Canadian couples generally, our soundings among those in touch with the research funding situation at the time this study was being planned convinced us that a modest beginning was the most feasible and appropriate goal to set for ourselves. We thus decided to restrict the study to Metropolitan Toronto, a city which is an important social system in its own right, as well as one which presents a varied social mosaic, both vertical and horizontal, that would provide the differentials in behaviour and attitude which are the picks and trowels of a sociological dig.

We are only too aware of the limitations placed on our ability to generalize about Canadian fertility as a result of this decision. Apart from the many regional variations which we miss, we are particularly disappointed not to be able to compare the views of Toronto couples with those of French-Canadian couples. We are pleased that this will soon be possible as a result of a recent study in Quebec undertaken by the demographers from the University of Montreal. These two studies taken together should further deepen our understanding of Canadian fertility although comparisons will be handicapped by differences in time periods. Plans are now being discussed for a national fertility survey which will signal the coming of age of demographic study in Canada.

As we put together the findings of this study we are cognizant of many questions left unanswered, often because the analysis involved ended in small numbers. It is our hope that our successes and failures will be studied closely in designing and executing the proposed national survey. Despite the strong cultural winds that blow across Canada's southern border there are certain distinctive aspects to Canadian fertility, some of which are revealed in this investigation. The strong pressures towards conformity with the content of other national surveys especially as the United Nations' World Population

Year, 1974, approaches should be balanced by the determination to explore what is unique to the couples of this country.

Perhaps a greater sacrifice than the restriction of geographic coverage was the decision to limit the investigation to women only—and to currently married women at that. This should be remedied in future investigations. No serious market researcher or political pollster would base his predictions of consumer or voter preferences on a single sex sample. Reproduction and the various forms of behaviour that attend it is even more of a dyadic relationship than buying a car or casting a vote.

In spite of these limitations on the size and scope of the study which we present more as a chronicle than a complaint, we believe that this study will be useful not merely as a forerunner of future studies, but as a source of information and suggestion for students of population and for those concerned with population as an object of public policy and programs. At the time this survey was undertaken there was very little official interest in population. That situation is rapidly changing. The data to be presented here on such things as family-size desires, on current and planned contraceptive behaviour, on attitudes towards abortion will, we believe, help to advance public understanding of the problem of population. We have intentionally refrained from a technical style of presentation in order to make the material useful to as wide a group of readers as possible.

The cooperation of many institutions and individuals made the study possible. The principal financial support was a major grant from the Canada Council which organization was also generous enough to provide two smaller continuation grants. Additional support was received from the University of Western Ontario and the Johns Hopkins University, mainly in the form of computer time and staff facilities. The book has been published with the help of a grant from the Social Science Research Council of Canada, using funds provided by the Canada Council.

The field work was done by Recon Research, Ltd., a private survey organization located in Toronto. The director, Mr. Brian Forrest, and his field staff were of great assistance in preparing the study for the field and in their expeditious handling of field problems. Dr. Ivan Fellegi helped in the design of the sample and preparation of the sampling frame. A number of persons have been involved in the various stages of processing and analysing of the data. Particular thanks are due to Roberta Ferrence, who supervised checking and coding of questionnaires and to Dorothy Worth of the University of Western Ontario and Judith Gehret of Johns Hopkins University who did most of the programming, and each in her individual way was of invaluable help in getting tabulations done through a series of ever-changing computer systems. Many students worked as research assistants at various stages and some used the data as thesis material. Here we would like to acknowledge the work of Rafiqul Huda Chaudhury, Harriett Destler, Freda Husic, John Kelly, Don Lavis, Pat Musson, Suzanne Myers, Trinidad Osteria, George Parakulam, Gordon Pinell, and Shan Ross.

Finally, we must thank our wives Ruth, Jane, and Nora for their patience and moral support during the years following the survey, when the authors were in three different locations trying to coordinate research and writing on the book.

T. R. Balakrishnan
J. F. Kantner
J. D. Allingham

1

Introduction

This is a study of the attitudes and behaviour of married women in Metropolitan Toronto concerning the past and prospective growth of their families. The basic information was collected in January–March 1968 through interviews with 1,632 wives in their reproductive years. The interviews dealt with a variety of topics: the number of births and miscarriages, the number of children wanted by the wife, the number she expected to have altogether, and the methods she has used or was using to avoid pregnancy. In addition, a wide variety of information on standard of living, religion, educational attainment, income, wife's labour force status, and ethnic and residential background were collected.

As the first large study of its kind in Canada it is hoped that the data will not only illuminate the nature of fertility in a major metropolitan community but may also provide some suggestions regarding Canadian fertility patterns which could be fruitfully investigated in a future national study.

Recent Fertility Trends in Canada

Soon after World War II, Canada experienced a sharp rise in fertility rates from its prewar levels, and crude birth rates remained around 28.0 per thousand population during the years 1946–56. However, since 1957 there has been a considerable decline in crude birth rates which reached an all time low of 17.4 per thousand in 1970.

Not only the crude rates, but more refined measures such as total fertility rates, general fertility rates, and legitimate fertility rates all show a steep decline in the last decade. The fairly steady marriage rates, around eight per thousand, and a slightly declining age at first marriage indicate that these fertility declines are not attributable to changing marriage patterns. The high rates immediately following World War II were in part caused by compressed birth intervals among young, recently married couples whose family building schedule had been set back by the war. The effect of these life cycle perturbations on fertility rates were attenuated by the late 1960s, as the post-war marriage cohorts completed their childbearing. The recent decline in the apparent absence of nuptiality changes suggests either a downward revision of norms regarding family size, or enhanced fertility control within the prevailing normative scheme or both. Henripin and Legare, for example, show that after controlling for changes in age–sex composition and nuptiality there still was a substantial decline in total and legitimate age specific fertility rates during the 1960s.[1]

The causes for this rapid decline in fertility rates must be sought in the attitudes of women towards family size, timing and spacing of births, and in their ability to achieve these desires through family limitation practices. As social norms and behaviour vary according to socio-economic characteristics, it is necessary to look at the various segments of the population. Detailed analytical studies on fertility behaviour are almost nonexistent in Canada. The few studies done using census materials, however, show significant differences in fertility performance by various characteristics such as ethnic origin, and religion.[2]

Apart from possible changes in social norms towards a smaller family size, a factor of importance during this period of rapid fertility decline is the emergence of oral contraception as a leading method of birth control. Through the data in this study we hope to shed some light on the factors contributing to current as well as expected fertility. We shall attempt to discover whether young married couples intend to have smaller families than those ten years earlier; what methods they use and expect to use to prevent pregnancy; and what basic conditions of family life influence attitudes towards family size, spacing between births, and birth control.

[1] See Henripin and Legare, "Recent Trends in Canadian Fertility."

[2] Henripin, *Trends and Factors of Fertility in Canada*; Krotki and Lapiere, "La fécondité au Canada selon la religion, l'origine ethnique et l'étât matrimonial."

Table 1 Fertility Rates for Canada, 1946–1970

Year	*Birth Rate per 1,000*	*Births per 1,000 Women in Ages 15–49*	*Total Fertility Rate*
1946	27.2	105.0	3,374
1947	28.9	112.4	3,595
1950	27.1	107.7	3,455
1955	28.2	116.5	3,831
1957	28.2	118.0	3,925
1959	27.4	116.3	3,935
1961	26.1	111.5	3,840
1963	24.6	105.3	3,669
1964	23.5	100.2	3,502
1965	21.3	90.3	3,145
1966	19.4	81.5	2,812
1967	18.2	75.8	2,586
1968	17.6	72.5	2,441
1969	17.6	71.7	2,388
1970	17.4	71.1	2,311

SOURCE: Vital Statistics of Canada annual reports.

Because of the lack of comparable Canadian research on the subject, reference to United States literature on fertility will often be made when we seek to put the Toronto data in broader perspective. National fertility surveys have been carried out in the United States every five years since 1955 providing a wealth of information on fertility and family planning. Canada, on the other hand, is only now discussing plans for the first country-wide survey.

The Sample

Interviews were conducted with 1,632 once married women under 46 years of age, currently living with their husbands in Metropolitan Toronto. Interviewees were selected in such a way as to constitute a scientific probability sample of approximately 300,000 Toronto wives who were estimated on the basis of the 1966 census to have the indicated characteristics at the time of the survey. Widows, divorcees, and wives not living with their husbands were not interviewed. Even though such women are a significant part of the female population in the reproductive years their impact on the birth rate is expected to be small. To observe these restrictions meant that approximately 5,243 households had to be contacted to yield 1,632 completed interviews with eligible respondents.

A two-stage sampling design was followed. First from a list of census enumeration areas from Metropolitan Toronto, 200 Enumeration Areas (E.A.'s) were selected with probabilities proportional to the number of married women in the E.A. as given in the 1966 census. For each selected E.A., a listing of all households was prepared using the city directory plus additional information where recent changes in land development had taken place. Sampling ratios for each E.A. were determined so as to yield approximately 12 eligible respondents per E.A. Using these sampling ratios households were selected systematically with a random start. A total of 5,243 households were contacted by telephone to obtain basic information on household composition needed to establish eligibility for the detailed interview. A few households in which the wife did not speak either English or Italian were excluded though other conditions of eligibility were fulfilled. At the initial design stage it was expected that such a design would yield 2,000 completed interviews allowing for refusals, those not at home, and so forth. However, the proportion of eligible respondents in sample households was somewhat lower than expected which resulted in a smaller number of completed interviews (1,632) than originally planned. Of the 2,023 eligible women, interviews were completed with 81 per cent. Some information on sample size and response rates are presented in table 2.

Though it would have been advisable to interview husbands as well, cost considerations ruled this out. However, some information on the husband was obtained from the wife.

The Interview

The respondents were interviewed by trained interviewers following a structured schedule. The schedule was pre-tested in London, Ontario with a sample of 150 respondents. The pre-test sample was chosen to represent the various segments of the population. The final interview schedule was a revised version of the pre-test schedule. The interviews averaged about one hour and fifteen minutes, varying in length from half an hour to as much as three hours. Both English and Italian versions of the questionnaire were employed.

Table 2 Distribution of Sample Households by Eligibility of Respondent and Response Rates

	Number	*Per Cent*
Total sample households	5,243	100.0
Eligible respondents	2,023	38.6
No eligible respondent	2,695	51.4
Refusals at initial contact	246	4.7
Loss due to language problems	120	2.3
Loss due to other causes	159	3.0
Eligible respondents	2,023	100.0
Interviewed	1,632	80.7
Not interviewed		
Refusals	234	11.5
Other	157	7.8

An important fact emerging from this investigation is that a vast majority of married women are willing to give to the best of their ability information about their family-planning practices and other highly personal topics in a direct interview situation.

In order to strike a balance between the routine description of fertility patterns and the more challenging job of analysing the data in search of explanations of such patterns we have adopted the practice of dividing each chapter into two parts: the first sections of each chapter are devoted simply to describing the findings with minimal attention to detailed analysis; the later sections contain more detailed statistical analysis and tests of various hypotheses.

2

Dimensions of Fertility

The level of fertility achieved by a couple is a function of many factors, such as values regarding family size, religious and other beliefs, knowledge and practice of birth control, financial situation, social identity, and reproductive capacity in biological terms. In this chapter we shall explore some of these relationships as they appear among the women in our sample.

Fecundity Impairment

A large number of women are unable to have the number of children they want because of fecundity impairment. While not all are definitely sterile, many of them can be classified as probably sterile on the basis of various health and medical indications. "Fecundity," or the capacity of a couple to have children in the future, is a hard concept to measure and no refined attempt is made in this study. As a crude approach, all women were asked: "Do you have any reasons to believe that you and your husband could not have another child if you wanted to?" and "If Yes, what is your reason for believing you can't have another child?"

Two hundred and nine women, or 12.8 per cent, said that they cannot have another child and an additional 32 women, or 2.0 per cent, were uncertain about their ability to conceive. Thus, the extent of sterility, including those who are probably sterile, was about 15 per cent of the total. However, only a fourth of these women were childless, that is, absolutely barren.[1] This would mean that out of the total group of infecund and subfecund women, three-fourths had become sterile after bearing one or more children. Part of this is attributable to voluntary sterilization. Because our sample is restricted to women currently living with their husbands, any generalization of the absolute infecundity observed to the general female population may be invalid. If infecundity selects against successful marriage, the level of infecundity in the general population could be higher than four per cent.

Operations for Health Reasons or to Prevent Contraception

About seven per cent of all women reported an operation either on themselves or on their husbands which made another pregnancy impossible. Of these 110 couples, the operation was on the woman in 98 cases and on the husband in 12 cases. Since we did not ask why the operation was performed it is not possible to separate those who had an operation for birth control purposes from those who had it for other reasons.

There was an increase in the percentage of sterilized women with an increase in number of pregnancies (table 3). Among women with three or fewer pregnancies the percentage was constant at five per cent, but among those who had four or more pregnancies the proportion varied from nine per cent for couples where the wife had four or five pregnancies to 20 per cent where the wife had six or more pregnancies.

As is to be expected, age of wife is positively associated with the probability of sterilization (table 4). Undoubtedly this is due to health reasons as well as to a desire to limit family size with increasing parity. There were proportionately very few couples who had an operation where the wife was less than 35 years of age. In the 35 and over group, 12 per cent were sterilized. One would expect on the basis of trends observed elsewhere that this percentage would increase in future. In the United States sterilization has shown a steady rise from nine per cent in the national survey of 1955 to 10 per cent in the 1960 and 14 per cent in the 1965 survey. By 1970 the percentage has increased further and sterilization has become the most prevalent method of birth control with couples in which the wife is 30 or over. This upward trend reflects a recent upsurge in vasectomies.

[1] In non-contraceptive populations, about four per cent of absolute infecundity is estimated. See Lorimer, *Culture and Human Fertility*, pp. 29-31.

Table 3 Percentage of Couples Who Had a Sterilizing Operation by Number of Pregnancies

Number of Pregnancies	*Percentage Who Had an Operation*	*Number of Couples in Base Group*
0	5	173
1	5	252
2–3	5	774
4–5	9	321
6 or more	20	112
Total	7	1632

Table 4 Percentage of Couples Who Had a Sterilizing Operation by Current Age of Wife

Wife's Current Age	*Percentage Sterilized Couples*	*Number of Couples in Base Group*
Less than 25	1	197
25–29	2	322
30–34	3	329
35–39	12	358
40 or more	12	426
Total	7	1632

Ideal, Desired, and Expected Family Size

One of the purposes of the survey was to determine the total number of children a couple is likely to have by the time childbearing is over. This expected completed family size tends to be a function of attitudes and desires towards family size, to the extent that these attitudes and desires are stable and to the extent that birth control is practised effectively. In this survey, information was obtained on three variables: the number of children a woman considers ideal for an average Canadian family, the number she actually desires herself, and the number she finally expects to have.

Differences between ideal and desired number of children are, at least conceptually, indications of discrepancies between general and personal norms about family size. The conceptual differences between these two measures have been emphasized by many researchers and their interrelationships have been analysed. Obviously actual performances may fall short or exceed these norms due to fecundity impairments, accidental pregnancies, conflicting attitudes of the partner, and other relevant factors. However imperfect, these measures of fertility preferences are assumed to have meaning as indications of the family-size goals couples would attempt to realize provided they knew how and were willing to meet the cost, psychic and otherwise, of so doing. Expected fertility is part preference and part perceived probability.

This section therefore presents data on ideal, desired, and expected number of children, the interrelationships between these three measures and their demographic correlates.

When 1,632 women were asked: "What would you regard as the ideal number of children for the average Canadian family?", 1,583 or 98 per cent gave numerical replies. An overwhelming majority reported two, three, or four children as ideal for an average Canadian family, with three being the most popular.

Desired number of children was determined by the question: "If you were to start married life over again, how many children in all would you want to have?"

Total expected family size was determined by adding the actual number of children a woman had at the time of the survey and the additional number she expected to have, the question asked being: "In addition to the children that you have, how many more do you intend to have?"

A slight modification of this question was put to pregnant women in order to make certain that they did not include their current pregnancy in their estimate of the number of additional children they expected.

In spite of some criticisms of its use to predict individual fertility, expected family size has come to be accepted as an important measure of future completed aggregate fertility which possesses considerable stability and reliability.[2] In addition, expectations regarding family size may be less sensitive to timing variations than are period fertility rates and thus changes in total expected family size are likely to reveal changes in family-size norms.

[2] Goldberg, Sharp, and Freedman, "The Stability and Reliability of Expected Family Size Data." Whelpton, Campbell, and Patterson, *Fertility and Family Planning in the U.S.*, p. 15. Freedman and Bumpass, "Fertility Expectations in the United States: 1962–1964." Ryder and Westoff, "The Trend of Expected Parity in the United States: 1955, 1960 and 1965."

The distribution of women by the three variables and parity are presented in table 5. Comparison of the means show that the ideal number (3.0) and the number desired (3.1) are similar. However, the expected number (2.8) is less than either the ideal or desired size. The most striking fact is the clear preference for 2–4 children and the avoidance of numbers below or above this range. We do not find the bimodality in the distribution of desired number which has been reported for the U.S. data.[3] There is less relative variation (S.D./mean) in the responses with respect to ideal and desired family size than with respect to expected or actual family size. This is not surprising since the perceptions of the general norm (ideal size) or its reflection in desired family size are more crystallized (smaller absolute and relative deviation—table 5) than either actual or expected fertility which reflect the idiosyncratic family formation paths followed by individual couples.

In common with other studies that have analysed the differences between these various hypothetical measures of completed fertility, we find that the number of children expected is less than the number considered as ideal or the number desired. With no subfecundity or infecundity and assuming perfect contraception, desired and expected fertility should be the same, provided the desired number is within the couple's means and provided there is no disagreement between husband and wife concerning reproductive goals. The fact that the expected number is lower than the number desired reflects the inability of some couples to have as many children as they want because of reproductive incapacity. For others who are fecund, the differences may reflect the fact that desires exceed expectation for want of social means. A simple tabulation of differences between desired and expected numbers by wife's education or by family income fails to show any consistent pattern. The tendency for desires to exceed expectations varies irregularly by family income, the differences being small in any case. Measured by education, desires exceed expectation by the greatest margin at the extremes of the educational scale.

These three measures are surrogates for completed family size and although each has its imperfections, they tend to point to the same conclusion: that the couples in our sample regard a figure close to three as the number they would like to have, expect to have, and

[3] Ryder and Westoff, *Reproduction in the United States, 1965*, p. 28. The bimodality observed in the U.S. data disappears when women of completed and incompleted fertility are analysed separately.

consider to be a good number generally. This observation, when combined with the mean number of children these couples have actually had (2.3), reveals that future childbearing will have to be confined to an average of less than one child per couple in order not to exceed the limits they have set for themselves. To put the matter in terms of the typical situation facing this group, given the average age of women in the sample and assuming that the risk of childbearing extends through age 45, the pregnancy rate that must be attained in order not to go beyond the desired number is approximately 12 per hundred woman years of exposure. This is well within the range of effectiveness of conventional methods of contraception. On the average, therefore, there appears to be no reason for women in this sample to exceed the number of children they desire. That a number will do so is to be expected since in speaking of average performance we recognize that some will exceed and some fall below the group mean.

The sharp boundaries which confine childbearing essentially to the range of two to four children are indicative of the operation of effective normative pressures which define a family of less than two children as "too small" and more than four as "too large."[4] Such compact distributions, especially with severe curtailment of the higher birth rates, are characteristic of modern populations with a high capacity for fertility regulation. By not being overly prescriptive and by being somewhat indifferent to variations in family size within the accepted range, the norm can accommodate different patterns of family formation. Those who are relatively well off can have somewhat larger families than others. But the differences cannot be great because great differences are not tolerated. We can see this in table 6 which shows that for a select subsample there is essential agreement on the number of children they would want to have if they were to do it again. The table also shows that there are differences in the number of children they have actually had, even when a good many factors affecting fertility are allowed for. What makes these findings interesting is that they refer to a group that presumably is able to actualize its desires (its members are both fecund and efficient at fertility regulation) and who, except for differences in their present situation (high, medium, or low relative income), would be similar in their reproductive performance. Assignment to a particular relative income category was made on the basis of a comparison of the husband's current income with the income that would be predicted for

[4] See Griffith, "Family Size Norms and Informal Social Control."

Table 5 Ideal, Desired, Total Expected, and Actual Number of Children

Number of Children	*Ideal*		*Desired*		*Expected*		*Actual*	
	N	%	*N*	%	*N*	%	*N*	%
0	3	.2	18	1.1	73	4.4	206	12.6
1	5	.3	20	1.3	120	7.3	300	18.4
2	538	33.8	542	34.2	553	33.9	509	31.2
3	558	35.0	474	29.9	463	28.4	332	20.3
4	434	27.2	419	26.5	275	16.9	166	10.2
5	33	2.1	43	2.7	81	5.0	68	4.2
6 or more	22	1.4	68	4.3	67	4.1	51	3.1
Total	1593	100.0	1584	100.0	1632	100.0	1632	100.0
Mean	3.01		3.07		2.82		2.26	
S.D.	.95		1.18		1.46		1.61	
S.D./Mean	.32		.38		.52		.71	

him on the basis of his age, education, and occupation.[5] In short, while those who can do so appear to adjust their fertility to their social and economic circumstances, with those in more favourable circumstances having more children, this is done within the narrow quantitative range of 2–4.[6]

Table 6 Unadjusted and Adjusted Mean Number of Children Ever Born and Desired, for a Native-Born Subsample *

	Mean Number of			
Relative	*Children Born*		*Children Desired***	
Income	*Unadjusted*	*Adjusted*	*Unadjusted*	*Adjusted*
	(1)	(2)	(3)	(4)
High	2.13	2.04	2.99	3.04
Medium	1.85	2.02	3.01	2.99
Low	1.89	1.89	3.01	2.95

**Couples who were native born, urbanites, presumably fecund, and who had never become pregnant while using contraception.*

***Number of children respondent would want if she could "start married life over again."*

N = 268 for columns 1 and 2 and 264 for columns 3 and 4. Adjustment in column 2 is made for the effect of husband's income, duration of marriage, age at marriage, wife's education, religion, her labour force status and work history; adjustment in column 4 is made for all of these variables, plus parity, husband's occupation, education, and wife's income.

Childbearing below the level required for population replacement is virtually excluded from consideration. Women who seek to establish careers with no involvement in motherhood are clearly marginal, and while our data do not reveal it directly, strong normative sanctions expressed by family, friends, and other agencies of social control define such a choice not only as marginal but also as deviant.[7] Transgressions into the higher zones of fertility are some-

[5] Chaudhury, "Relative Income and Fertility."

[6] Cumulative fertility is of course achieved over time. Thus a classification of relative income based on present circumstances may be invalid for earlier periods. However, a calculation of relative income at the time of marriage when related to the mean interval from marriage to first birth (excluding apparent premarital conceptions) shows that an inverse relationship exists (table 7).

[7] See Griffith, *Family Size Norms and Informal Social Control.* While Griffith's data are taken from a national sample of the U.S. population, the same social dynamics no doubt have been operative on the women in our sample.

what less exceptional and probably regarded as less deviant than the failure to cross the two-child threshhold. The likelihood that the lower normative bond is maintained by strong negative sanctions against voluntary childlessness and the decision to have an "only child," is apt to be as much of an obstacle to female "liberation" as discriminating hiring practices or the pervasive manifestation of "male chauvinism."[8]

Table 7 Unadjusted and Adjusted Mean Number of Years from Marriage to First Birth by Relative Income at Time of Marriage *

Relative Income at Marriage	*Mean Interval in Years* Unadjusted	*Adjusted***
High	2.8	2.9
Medium	3.1	3.3
Low	3.7	3.4

**Native born urban women, all of whom conceived after marriage and who never had an accidental conception.*

***Adjusted for: duration of marriage, age at marriage, present relative income, income at marriage, husband's income and education, wife's education, and husband's former occupation.*

N = 218

Some further insight into the data on the expected number is obtained by comparing it with the size of completed family that can be calculated from the application of estimated parity progression ratios (see chapter 4). The average number of children so estimated is 3.25 in contrast to 2.82, the mean number expected. Thus, if the women in our sample were to repeat the experience of those who in a sense have preceded them, their completed family size would be 15 per cent larger than the one they expect to have. It seems reasonable to infer from this that there is in progress some downward revision of family-size norms.

The distributions show considerable variation. While for ideal family size, 96 per cent gave answers of two to four, there is progressively greater variation in desired, expected, and current fertility as revealed by the standard deviations. As many of the women in

[8] Granted that the normative pattern of childbearing itself is a reflection of a limited set of legitimate female roles, the significant fact is that the pattern is expressed by our respondents who are women.

our sample will be having additional children, actual or current fertility is not strictly comparable with the other three measures of family size which focus on completed family size.

Differences in ideal, desired, and expected family size are also found when characteristics such as age and religion are considered (table 8). Mean ideal and desired number of children show a tendency to rise with age, both for Protestants and Catholics. The fact that this rise with age parallels the rise in actual fertility raises the possibility that the hypothetical responses are to some extent rationalizations of actual experience. There is no satisfactory way within the limits of these data to overcome this problem. However, it is interesting to recall that, as noted earlier in comparing expected fertility with completed fertility estimated from parity progression ratios, there is some evidence to suggest that fertility norms may be falling. To the extent this is true we may have confidence in the trends by age in ideal and desired fertility. Also consistent with the view that the upward trend of desired fertility with age is not wholly a rationalization of actual fertility is the fact that expected fertility does not vary with age in any uniform way. Thus older women do not desire larger families because they expect their families to be larger than the average. Rather, they desire larger families than they expect to have.

Relative differences in the three measures are very similar within religious groups. However, there are substantial and consistent differences between religious groups overall and within each age group.

Interrelations between Ideal, Desired, and Expected Family Size

Comparisons of mean values show general differences but do not reveal the extent of relationship between the various measures for individual women. The closeness of responses are measured in this section by reliability ratios as first used by Ryder and Westoff.[9] The procedure involves taking the numbers giving the same responses to each pair of questions and then reducing them by the numbers who would be expected to give the same response if there was no relationship between the two variables. This number is divided by the total number less the number expected to give the same responses. Symbolically, the ratio is defined as O–E/N–E where O is the observed number of cases in the equality diagonal, E is the number of cases expected in the equality diagonal under the assumption of randomness and N is the total number of cases. Under a perfect relationship, that is where all the responses are the same, all cases will be on the

[9] Ryder and Westoff, *Reproduction in the United States*, p. 29.

equality diagonal, the value of O will be N and the ratio will be unity. Under no relationship the value of O will be E and the ratio will be zero.

Table 8 Mean Ideal, Desired, and Expected Family Size by Religion and Age of Wife

Religion and Age of Wife	*Number of Women*	*Mean Ideal*	*Number of Children Desired*	*Number of Children Expected*
Protestant				
18–24	108	2.78	2.66	2.70
25–29	195	2.74	2.85	2.65
30–34	188	2.71	2.76	2.65
35–39	222	2.95	3.09	2.88
40 or more	261	3.08	3.10	2.59
Total	974	2.88	2.95	2.69
Catholic				
18–24	62	3.06	3.18	2.88
25–29	102	3.11	3.11	2.98
30–34	111	3.28	3.34	3.30
35–39	102	3.20	3.30	2.98
40 or more	121	3.46	3.56	3.17
Total	498	3.25	3.32	3.10
Others				
18–24	27	2.95	3.17	2.84
25–29	24	3.04	2.83	2.76
30–34	30	2.87	2.97	2.61
35–39	33	3.11	2.83	2.69
40 or more	44	3.14	3.18	2.68
Total	158	3.04	3.00	2.70
GRAND TOTAL	1630	3.01	3.07	2.82

The highest relationship is between current fertility and total expected children and between ideal and desired number of children. The former is not surprising as current cumulative fertility is a large fraction of the expected number. The high ratio between the ideal and desired number indicates that for a large portion of women the ideal family size they prescribe for others is also the size desired for themselves. One might expect if the idea of the "average Canadian family" conjured up the same general picture in the minds of our respondents and if they differentiated between the norms to which they subscribed and the norms they prescribed for others, that the difference between "ideal" and "desired" values would increase as one approaches the extremes of the socio-economic scale. This, however, turns out not to be the case. The great majority, somewhere between two-thirds and three-fourths of the respondents, regardless of education, occupation, income, religion, or duration of marriage give the same number in response to both questions. This probably results from a general tendency to see oneself as average.

Table 9 Correspondence between Different Measures of Family Size

Family Size Measures	*Ratio**
Ideal/desired	.60
Ideal/expected	.31
Ideal/current	.12
Desired/expected	.40
Desired/current	.16
Current/expected	.62

**Ratio approaches 1 if both measures of family size are the same; e.g., if there is correspondence between ideal and desired family size. Allowance is made for some randomness in response thereby assuming that some correspondence could be fortuitous thus depressing the calculated value of the ratio below the simple ratio of observed responses.*

There is no doubt that the two concepts of ideal and desired number function somewhat independently of each other. Respondents who desire two, three, or four children, that is, those whose preferences fall within the widely endorsed normative range, give the same number as the ideal. Above and below this range, however, the identity between desired and ideal values is broken. Almost all persons who desire less than two children put the ideal number for an average Canadian family at two or above. Conversely, two-thirds of those whose desired number of children exceeds the two to four range see the ideal size as something smaller. That the two concepts are mutually interactive is also evident in that the regression of ideal values towards the two–four range, in those instances where desired values fall outside the range, tends to be to the nearest value within the range. Thus most persons who desire less than two children put the ideal number at the lower end of the two–four range. Those who desire five or more put the ideal number towards the higher end of the range.

The low ratios shown in table 9 for expected number with either ideal or desired number is an indication of the difficulties that face many couples in attaining their family size preferences. Implied in this is the tendency noted earlier for desires to outrun expectations.

Group Differences in Family Size

Differences in the fertility of various religious, social, and economic groups result from differences in the number of children desired and the willingness and ability to control fertility to achieve this desire. In Canada, substantial differences in fertility by religion, type of residence, country of birth, education, and income of husband are reported by Henripin in an analysis of 1961 census information.[10] While these findings are significant they cannot depict trends in fertility differentials. Moreover, census data provide information only on past reproductive behaviour and nothing about future expectations of couples who have not completed their families. In a rapidly changing society these expectations are crucial for predicting future fertility patterns. In the past, Canadian fertility trends and differentials have been similar to those in the United States with an apparent time lag of a few years. Thus, in the absence of detailed fertility studies, there has been a tendency to accept the findings for the United States as generally valid for Canada. Given the socio-cultural differences between the two countries this is a patently undependable base for an understanding of Canadian fertility.

In this section we shall examine the number of children that women had at the time of the survey and the total number they expect to have by the time they are through with childbearing. We shall be interested in finding differences in these measures of fertility by religion, education, income, wife's labour force status, husband's occupation, and nativity. Some attention is given also to the number of children regarded as ideal and the number desired.

Religion

The most important religious differences in actual fertility and future expectations stem from the differing attitudes and values of Protestants and Catholics. The greater fertility of Catholics has been

[10] Henripin, *Trends and Factors of Fertility in Canada.*

attributed to the teaching of the Church that the primary purpose of marriage is procreation, in contrast to the Protestant church which tacitly permits avoidance or postponement of childbearing for a number of social and economic considerations. Canadian Catholic fertility has consistently been higher than non-Catholic fertility in the past. Using 1941 and 1961 census data on children ever born to women in the reproductive ages, Henripin concludes that for the 20–year period Catholic–non-Catholic differentials in fertility have been remarkably constant.[11] As religious differences are often confounded with differences in income, education of wife, and type of residence, Henripin controls for these factors and still finds that Catholic fertility which was about 28 per cent higher in 1941 remained at about the same high level in 1961. Subsequent to this period there were important innovations in contraceptive techniques such as the oral pill combined with the ambiguities Catholics experienced regarding the pill until the Church's position was clarified in late 1968. In spite of these developments some have conjectured that Catholic fertility is likely to remain higher than non-Catholic fertility.[12]

The absence of time-trend data on fertility attitudes in Canada makes the evaluation of changes in family-size desires by religion impossible. However, in the United States, looking at the data collected in national surveys over more than two decades since World War II, Blake concludes that the ideal family-size desires of Catholics and non-Catholics have been converging. In spite of the Church's unchanged position encouraging large families, "lay Catholics are generally further from sharing their Church's views concerning family size than they are from sharing those of non-Catholics."[13] It should be interesting to investigate differences in ideal family-size desires by religion as these would indicate future trends in fertility especially if Catholics tend to adopt more efficient contraceptive methods in the future.

We will look at some of the fertility differentials by religion and in the subsequent sections examine the confounding effects of other factors such as education, income, wife's labour force status, and occupation of the husband on these religious differences.

The average number of births to women by the time of the survey was 2.25, with the Catholics having a higher mean of 2.51 compared

[11] Henripin, *Trends and Factors of Fertility in Canada*, p. 211.
[12] Henripin, *Trends and Factors of Fertility in Canada*, p. 212.
[13] Judith Blake, "Americanization of Catholic Reproductive Ideals."

to 2.14 for the Protestants. The total expected number of births by the end of the reproductive period was 3.10 for the Catholics and 2.69 for the Protestants. In the earlier national surveys done in the United States the differences between Catholics and Protestants actually increased during the period 1955–1965. It should be emphasized, however, that the Toronto sample is not strictly comparable with the United States sample which includes both rural and urban women. If only metropolitan United States couples are compared the differences should not be great as the urban fertility is generally lower than rural fertility.

The differences between actual and expected family size for the Toronto sample are almost the same for all religious groups. In the earlier surveys done in the United States (though not strictly comparable due to the urban nature of our sample) the differences between actual and expected fertility were not the same for the various religious groups. Differences between the actual and expected fertility of non-Catholics do not show any particular time trend in the United States data, and are similar to comparable differences found in the Canadian data. For Catholics, however, it is a more complicated case. Regardless of the level of actual fertility, Catholics in the U.S. have on the average expected an additional one or more children whereas among the group of Canadian Catholics the expected increment in family size is only about half as great. An interpretation of this is that the Canadian women are more confident of their ability to regulate future fertility. Consistent with this is the much greater prevalence of oral contraception among our Canadian couples than has been true of the Catholics in the U.S. surveys reported here.[14]

Comparison of expected family size with the number of children considered ideal for the average Canadian family and also comparison with the number women would like to have if they could live their lives again, shows that the total expected is likely to be lower than both the ideal and desired family sizes for all the religious groups and for Protestants and Catholics by about the same amount (table 10). The differences between expected and either ideal or

[14] Very recent surveys in the United States show that there has been a profound decline in actual and expected number of births especially in the younger cohorts. Actual births for age group 18-24 in 1972 was only 0.9 with an expected total of 2.3 compared with 1.5 and 3.1 reported for this age group in the 1965 national survey. This may mean much higher use of oral contraception. See U.S. Department of Commerce, *Birth Expectations and Fertility, June 1972.*

desired number is much greater in our sample than is found in the most recent national survey done in the United States.[15]

Religiosity as measured by Church attendance has a positive relationship to fertility both for Protestants and for Catholics (table 11). Regular churchgoers have higher fertility expectations and generally had more children at the time of the interview. The relationship appears to be as strong for Protestants as for Catholics, a finding that is at variance with similar studies done in the United States. Freedman *et al.* in their 1955 Growth of American Families study conclude that among Protestants, church attendance makes little difference, but among the Catholics, substantial differences exist.[16] Among Toronto Protestant women, total expected family size for those who do not attend church was 2.59 as against 3.02 for those who attend Church five or more times in an "average fall or winter month." For Catholics, the comparable figures are 2.93 and 3.21, a smaller absolute as well as relative difference. Whereas among Protestants increases in frequency of attendance are fairly regularly associated with an increase in fertility, Catholics exhibit a threshhold at a level of three or four times per month.

Catholics exceed Protestants at each age in both the average number of children and in the total number they expect to have (table 12). The relationship of total expected to age is erratic, with Catholic women aged 30–34 having the highest expectations, whereas it is among Protestant women aged 35–39 that the highest expectations are found. Looking at the total number of children expected in relation to the number already born, we note that among women under 30, Catholics do not expect to have a larger number of additional births than do Protestants. This has the interesting implication that their control of fertility will have to be as effective as that of their Protestant sisters if their expectations are to be fulfilled. In other words, the ultimate expected family size of Catholic women is more like that of Protestant women than their accumulated fertility up to the time of the survey. A variant on this observation is to note that the total expectations of the youngest group of Protestant women is slightly above (2.70 vs. 2.56) the average number born to Protestant

[15] Ryder and Westoff, *Reproduction in the United States, 1965*, pp. 22-28. For white women the values are as follows: expected, 3.28; ideal, 3.24; desired, 3.29. Here again more recent surveys show less difference. See U.S. Department of Commerce, *Birth Expectations and Fertility, June 1972*.

[16] Freedman, *et al.*, *Family Planning, Sterility and Population Growth*, pp. 201-83.

Table 10 Ideal, Desired, and Total Expected Number of Children by Religion of Wife

Religion of Wife	*Number of Wives*	*Mean Number of Children*			*Differences*	
		Ideal	*Desired*	*Expected*	*Ideal Minus Expected*	*Desired Minus Expected*
Protestants	973	2.88	2.95	2.69	.19	.26
Catholics	498	3.25	3.32	3.10	.15	.22
Other	159	3.04	3.00	2.70	.34	.30
Total	1630	3.01	3.07	2.82	.19	.25

Table 11 Mean Number of Actual and Expected Births for Protestants and Catholic Wives by Frequency of Wife's Church Attendance

Monthly Church Attendance	*Protestants*			*Catholics*		
		Births			*Births*	
	Women	*Actual*	*Expected*	*Women*	*Actual*	*Expected*
Does not attend	407	2.06	2.59	73	2.47	2.93
Twice or less	309	2.09	2.72	124	2.40	2.94
3 or 4 times	175	2.27	2.70	198	2.58	3.20
5 or more times	82	2.59	3.02	103	2.53	3.23
Total	973	2.15	2.69	498	2.51	3.10

women 40 and over who have largely completed their childbearing. Young Catholic women on the other hand intend to finish with fewer children (2.88 vs. 3.13) than Catholics aged 40 and above have had.

Table 12 Mean Number of Actual and Expected Births by Religion and Age of Wife

Age and Religion of Wife	*Number of Wives*	*Actual Births*	*Expected Births*	*Additional Expected*
Age 18–24				
Protestants	108	.85	2.70	1.85
Catholics	62	1.26	2.88	1.62
Others	27	1.17	2.84	1.67
Age 25–29				
Protestants	195	1.36	2.65	1.29
Catholics	102	1.75	2.98	1.23
Others	24	1.64	2.76	1.12
Age 30–34				
Protestants	188	2.30	2.65	.35
Catholics	111	2.89	3.30	.41
Others	30	1.94	2.61	.67
Age 35–39				
Protestants	222	2.69	2.88	.19
Catholics	102	2.72	2.98	.26
Others	33	2.47	2.69	.22
Age 40 or more				
Protestants	261	2.56	2.59	.03
Catholics	121	3.13	3.17	.04
Others	44	2.55	2.68	.03
Total	1630	2.25	2.82	.57

A tabulation by duration of marriage (table 13) even without a direct age control again shows many of the same patterns as were noted in the analysis by age above: Catholic fertility and total expectations are consistently higher and recently married couples have completed family-size expectations that fall below the levels achieved by women whose fertility is completed. Again, the difference in this respect is slight for Protestants (2.59 vs. 2.83) but for Catholics it is even more evident (3.12 vs. 3.65) than was the case for age. If duration groups are combined, say those under ten years and those of 11 or more years, in order to increase the number of cases in the comparison, we find again that the actual fertility of women in the high duration group is greater than the total expected fertility of women married less than ten years. This could be due either to a downward revision of the family-size norm or to excess fertility among women of longer marital duration, to invalid projections of expected fertility on the part of young women, or to some combination of these.

Education and Income

Differences in the average number of children by education are for both Protestants and Catholics compounds of possible education effects and differences in age—the less educated being somewhat older on the average. There is, therefore, less ambiguity and greater interest in the data on total expectations. These indicate that among Catholics the highest expectation is given by those with the highest education whereas among Protestants and other religious groups the reverse is true (table 14). However, the number of college-educated Catholics is small and thus these results should not be over-interpreted. As we shall see in a later chapter, better-educated Catholics have been less inclined to use contraception than less-educated Catholics and among those who have used contraception the better educated have shown greater partiality towards the rhythm method. They were also relatively late as a group in accepting oral contraception although by the time of the survey they had surpassed less educated Catholics in the use of oral contraception. Despite this history of below average use, the better-educated Catholics have had fewer births than less-educated Catholics. Thus their relatively high total expected fertility would not seem to reflect a lack of confidence in their ability to regulate their fertility but rather a real preference for more children.

The analysis by income (table 15) without control for age also presents problems of interpretation since income and age are, to a degree, positively correlated. Thus the tendency for the average number of births to the time of interview to increase with income for both Protestants and Catholics is perhaps influenced by age. The total expected family size does not vary with income in any readily interpretable fashion for any of the religious groups. Perhaps the significance of this observation lies in the implications for theories that assume the "demand" for children to be income elastic. Becker, the original proponent of an economy theory of fertility based on the theory of consumer behaviour, suggested treating children as a consumption good analogous to cars, houses, and refrigerators. There is an income elasticity with respect to quality and quantity of children and it is likely to be positive. In other words, the larger the income

Table 13 Mean Number of Actual and Expected Births by Religion and Duration of Marriage

Religion and Duration of Marriage	*Number of Wives*	*Actual Births*	*Expected Births*	*Additional Expected*
Less than 3 years				
Protestants	85	.32	2.59	2.27
Catholics	33	.52	3.12	2.60
3–5 years				
Protestants	100	1.03	2.49	1.41
Catholics	59	1.37	2.97	1.60
6–10 years				
Protestants	208	1.90	2.56	.66
Catholics	133	2.29	2.84	.55
11–15 years				
Protestants	251	2.64	2.80	.16
Catholics	125	2.81	3.02	.21
16–20 years				
Protestants	187	2.70	2.72	.02
Catholics	102	3.22	3.37	.15
More than 20 years				
Protestants	143	2.80	2.83	.03
Catholics	46	3.65	3.65	.00
Total	1632	2.25	2.82	.57

the larger the desired family size is likely to be.[17] This position has been severely attacked by some demographers, especially Blake who points out the limited relevance of the consumer durable analogy and the importance of social norms, familial goals, and other social factors in the influence of desire for children.[18] Further modifications to the Becker model have been suggested by Easterlin and Namboodiri to take account of some of these criticisms. They emphasize the importance of introducing a time-orientation, such as income at various points of time in the life cycle, opportunity costs to parents, and the

[17] Becker, "An Economic Analysis of Fertility." Economic formulations such as Becker's escape easy refutation by evidence such as we have presented by suggesting that "quality" can be substituted for quantity. Thus what we would need would be total expenditures for childbearing rather than the mere quantity of children ever born.

[18] Blake, "Are Babies Consumer Durables?" Ryder, "Comments."

necessity of considering each parity separately in a utility analysis.[19] It is not our purpose here to go into a detailed discussion of the economic analysis of fertility but to alert the reader to the difficulties in arriving at a valid conclusion on the relationship between income and fertility. Our analysis here is restricted to only one point of time, namely at the time of the survey, and this measure of income does not support the hypothesis that income is directly related to family size.

Table 14 Mean Number of Actual and Expected Births by Religion and Education of Wife

Religion and Education of Wife	*Number of Wives*	*Actual Births*	*Expected Births*
Protestants			
Less than 8 years	100	2.84	3.02
High School 1–3 years	412	2.24	2.69
High School 4–5 years	330	1.97	2.54
College*	131	1.81	2.79
Total	973	2.15	2.69
Catholics			
Less than 8 years	219	2.61	3.00
High School 1–3 years	142	2.57	3.14
High School 4–5 years	105	2.22	3.11
College*	32	2.51	3.56
Total	498	2.51	3.10
Other Religions			
Less than 8 years	43	2.56	2.84
High School 1–3 years	47	2.29	2.79
High School 4–5 years	41	1.78	2.56
College*	27	1.65	2.56
Total	158	2.11	2.70

**College includes those who had some university education, those who earned a degree, and those who had an education in nursing or teaching.*

19 Easterlin, "Toward a Socio-Economic Theory of Fertility." Namboodiri, "Some Observations on the Economic Framework for Fertility Analysis."

Table 15 Mean Number of Actual and Expected Births by Religion and Income of Husband

Religion of Wife and Income of Husband	*Number of Wives*	*Actual Births*	*Expected Births*
Protestants			
Less than $4000	50	1.62	2.76
$4000–$5999	199	2.20	2.80
$6000–$7999	258	1.96	2.59
$8000–$9999	152	2.06	2.68
$10000–$11999	130	2.17	2.51
$12000 or more	129	2.67	2.91
Total	918	2.15	2.69
Catholics			
Less than $4000	48	2.38	3.33
$4000–$5999	173	2.35	3.02
$6000–$7999	117	2.48	3.11
$8000–$9999	54	2.51	3.02
$10000–$11999	36	2.86	3.00
$12000 or more	24	2.83	3.29
Total	452	2.51	3.10
Other Religions			
Less than $4000	14	2.29	3.07
$4000–$5999	45	2.22	2.56
$6000–$7999	19	2.05	3.06
$8000–$9999	22	1.91	2.73
$10000–$11999	14	1.86	2.36
$12000 or more	28	2.21	2.57
Total	142	2.11	2.70

The complete lack of overlap in the expectations of Protestants and Catholics, regardless of their income levels, is the truly important fact to be noted in these data. It reaffirms the significance of religion as a determinant of gross fertility differentials.

Wife's Labour Force Status

Substantial differences in fertility exist between women in the labour force and women not in the labour force, in all religious groups. Not only actual fertility but total expected fertility was higher among women who were not in the labour force compared to women in the labour force, among both Protestants and Catholics (table 16). Labour force participation is of course related to other socio-economic variables like education and income, and moreover is, to some extent, selective of low fertility women. That it has independent significance apart from these interrelationships is scarcely contestable.

Most analysis of the interrelationship of female employment and fertility has dealt with the simple working–non-working dichotomy. A woman's work history may be integrated with childbearing in a variety of ways so that it is essential to look at the process with respect to life-cycle segments. To be a member of the labour force has more bearing on fertility at some periods of marriage and at some stages of family building than at others. Recent discussions have recognized this point and have laid particular stress on the nature of work experience in early marriage. The argument is that alternatives to motherhood and domesticity are more readily adopted if early childbearing is deferred in favour of full-time employment. This permits the formation of tastes and habits that have a long-term influence on family formation. This thesis was investigated among a subsample of women who were neither premaritally pregnant nor subfecund and whose husbands worked full time at the time of their marriage thus alleviating the pressure of work in order to substitute for the husband's income.[20] The results shown in table 17 indicate that early work experience is significantly related to the mean number of expected children when the period of employment exceeds ten years. Shorter work periods appear to make relatively little difference on expected fertility. An attempt to classify the wife's occupation qualitatively, that is in terms of the skill and education required and thus its presumed inherent satisfaction, produced mixed results in so far as expected family size was concerned.

Husband's Occupation

Fertility differentials associated with husband's occupation seem somewhat clearer than in the case of income (table 18). Women whose husbands are in the higher status occupations such as the professions and managerial positions have present fertility and future expected fertility similar to blue-collar workers. Lower white-collar groups have the lowest fertility expectations. This U shaped pattern

[20] This analysis was carried out by Harriet P. Destler, and is more fully described in her master's thesis, "Work Before the First Birth: Its Relation to Fertility and Contraceptive Practice." The analysis was confined to women born in Canada, the United States, or the United Kingdom.

Table 16 Mean Number of Actual and Expected Births by Religion and Labour Force Participation of Wife

Religion and Wife's Labour Force Status	*Number of Wives*	*Actual Births*	*Expected Births*
Protestants			
In Labour Force	355	1.67	2.45
Not in Labour Force	619	2.43	2.83
Total	974	2.15	2.69
Catholics			
In Labour Force	182	2.11	2.76
Not in Labour Force	316	2.73	3.30
Total	498	2.51	3.10
Other Religions			
In Labour Force	47	1.68	2.51
Not in Labour Force	111	2.30	2.78
Total	158	2.11	2.70

Table 17 Mean Number of Actual and Expected Births by Duration of Employment before First Birth *

Estimated Work Experience Prior to First Birth	*Number of Wives*	*Actual Births*	*Number of Wives*	*Expected Births*
0–4 years	139	2.35	136	3.06
5–10 years	437	2.26	422	2.98
More than 10 years	231	1.88	220	2.35
Total	807	2.17	778	2.82

**Limited to respondents who were not premaritally pregnant; who were not subfecund at time of survey; whose husbands worked full time at marriage; and who were born in Canada, the United States, or the United Kingdom.*

obtains in all religious groups. The highest expected total fertility is found among upper white-collar Catholics. Their expectation of 3.27 children is substantially higher than 2.84 for lower white-collar Catholics. Some of this difference is probably attributable to their higher educational levels but in the absence of control for education and age, the independent effect of occupation is hard to assess.

Table 18 Mean Number of Actual and Expected Births by Religion of Wife and Occupation of Husband

Religion of Wife and Occupation of Husband	*Number* of Wives*	*Actual Births*	*Expected Births*
Protestants			
Upper white collar	423	2.22	2.71
Lower white collar	195	1.95	2.57
Blue collar	350	2.22	2.73
All Protestants	973	2.15	2.69
Catholics			
Upper white collar	121	2.72	3.27
Lower white collar	65	2.14	2.84
Blue collar	307	2.52	3.07
All Catholics	498	2.51	3.10
Other Religions			
Upper white collar	72	1.82	2.74
Lower white collar	24	2.04	2.54
Blue collar	61	2.48	2.72
All other religions	158	2.11	2.70

**Small discrepancies in totals are due to item non-response.*

Nativity

Nativity as a factor in differential fertility has been losing ground in postwar research. In the first of the national fertility studies in the United States conducted in 1955, Freedman and others justify the dropping of nativity by pointing out the virtual disappearance of differentials by 1950 in the age specific fertility rates of native-born white with all white women in the United States.[21] The later national studies also fail to publish data by nativity.[22] The general assumption is that because of a decrease in the foreign-born population and because of a narrowing of differentials, nativity is no longer important.

However, some recent evidence seems to indicate a re-emergence and, indeed, a reversal of differentials in fertility by nativity. The

[21] Freedman, *et al., Family Planning, Sterility and Population Growth*, pp. 422-23. This does not include native Indians or Mexican Americans who have substantially higher fertility than persons with European background.

[22] Whelpton, *et al., Fertility and Family Planning in the United States.*

substantially higher fertility of foreign-born women in the early decades of this century vanished by the middle of the century, but since then there seems to be a trend towards lower fertility among foreign-born women. Bogue, looking at 1960 census data, points out that ever-married, foreign-born white women had lower fertility than comparable native-born whites for all ages under 55 years of age, and speculated that recent migrants from Europe may be bringing with them the European pattern of lower fertility.[23]

For Canada, 1961 census data show that fertility of foreign-born women was considerably lower than that of native-born women as can be seen from table 19. The number of children born per 1,000 ever-married women was lower for the foreign born in all the age groups. Generally lower fertility among foreign-born women and considerable differences among them according to country of birth has also been noticed by other students of Canadian fertility.[24]

The Canadian differences are greater than the comparable U.S. differences, since the native-born Canadian women had higher fertility than native-born United States women whereas the foreign born in the two countries had about the same level of fertility.

Foreign-born women in our sample consituted 40 per cent of the total. This is much higher than the national figure and indicates the heavy immigration into Toronto in the last decade. As can be seen from the data in table 20, foreign-born women, both among Protestants and Catholics, had lower actual and total expected fertility. The age and marriage duration distributions of foreign-born women were very similar to native-born women, indicating that the causes are socio-economic rather than demographic.

To better understand the behaviour of foreign-born women, they were further classified into four groups according to the region of their country of birth: Western Europe, Eastern Europe, Mediterranean, and Other. The majority of foreign-born women were married to foreign-born men, the percentage married to native-born men being only 25.2 per cent for Western Europe, 11.8 per cent for Eastern Europe, and a mere 3.2 per cent for Mediterranean women.

The variations in actual and total expected fertility are fairly clear cut among the various categories of foreign-born women. Women born in Western Europe have the lowest actual and expected fertility followed in ascending order by women born in Eastern Europe and

[23] Bogue, *Principles of Demography*, pp. 696-97.

[24] Henripin, *Trends and Factors of Fertility in Canada*, pp. 153-54. Krotki and Lapierre, "La fécondité au Canada selon la religion, l'origine ethnique et l'étât matrimonial."

the Mediterranean. The group shown in table 21 as "other" represents a diverse mixture of national origins. Because of this, and because of their relatively small number (N=72) little attention is given them in this analysis. Canadian-born women display the highest expected fertility even though their actual fertility by 1968 is somewhat lower than women from Mediterranean countries.

Table 19 Number of Children Born per 1000 Ever-Married Women 15 Years or Older by Nativity, Canada 1961 *

Age of Mother	*Native Born*	*Foreign Born*
15–19	756	511
20–24	1,378	1,000
25–29	2,288	1,611
30–34	2,921	2,156
35–39	3,264	2,495
40–44	3,346	2,541
45–49	3,191	2,508
50–54	3,288	2,614

**Calculated from 1961 Census figures D.B.S.* Census of Canada, *Bulletin 4–1–7, tables G2 and G3.*

With respect to "ideal" and "desired" family size, the order by nativity is the same as that found with respect to expected family size. Western European women consider the ideal family as one slightly less than three children; all other groups state an ideal just above three. Overall, the range of differences was quite small. Somewhat greater differences are observed for "desired" family size. Women from Western and Eastern Europe set their desires slightly below their notion of the "ideal" number. In the case of all other groups, desires outrun ideals by a small margin. Canadian-born women desire larger families than any of the major immigrant blocks.

Comparison of actual fertility at the time of the survey and total expected fertility reveals the interesting fact that the additional number of births expected varies around 0.5 and is nearly the same for all groups. With a mean age fairly close to 34, these women have on an average about eleven remaining years of reproductive life. At least for those not practising effective contraception, one wonders whether the final completed fertility might not exceed expectations.

Table 20 Mean Number of Actual and Expected Births by Religion and Nativity of Wife

Religion and Nativity of Wife	*Number of Wives*	*Actual Births*	*Expected Births*
Protestants			
Native born	692	2.20	2.75
Foreign born	282	2.04	2.53
Total	974	2.15	2.69
Catholics			
Native born	205	2.58	3.30
Foreign born	293	2.46	2.97
Total	498	2.51	3.10
All Religions			
Native born	958	2.28	2.89
Foreign born	674	2.22	2.75
Total	1632	2.26	2.82

Table 21 Mean Number of Actual, Expected, and Desired Births by Nativity of Wife

	Country of Birth					
Number of Births	*Canada*	*Western Europe*	*Eastern Europe*	*Mediterranean*	*Other*	*Total*
Actual	2.29	2.02	2.18	2.35	2.47	2.25
Expected	2.92	2.54	2.60	2.85	3.29	2.84
Desired	3.05	2.83	3.02	3.04	3.15	3.01
Number of wives	917	290	102	155	72	1536

An examination within nativity groups by such variables as religion, education, and income yields results in the expected direction. Women born in Western Europe who are predominantly Protestant (70 per cent), well educated, and have relatively high incomes, have low fertility. Eastern European-born women who are about 43 per cent Catholic, less educated, and with lower incomes have somewhat higher fertility. Finally, the Mediterranean women who are 80 per cent Roman Catholic, 84 per cent with less than ninth grade education, and 64 per cent with less than $6,000 annual income, have the highest fertility. Among the native born, the classic pattern of socio-economic variation is less pronounced. They have higher fertility in spite of higher income and a greater percentage of Protestants. This would seem to indicate the probable influence of other factors such as general economic prosperity and changing family role structure.

The lower fertility of foreign-born women and the differences among them according to ethnicity is an important finding. Because of small numbers when classification is made by country of birth, this line of analysis is not pursued in depth. However, some controls for nativity are made whenever feasible in later chapters. Given the importance of immigration and the ethnic factor in Canadian fertility it would be advisable in future fertility research to give these variables greater consideration in the planning stage itself, something we were not able to foresee in our study.

Summary

Comparisons of ideal, desired, and expected fertility show that completed family size, as estimated by the respondent, is likely to fall short of either the ideal or desired numbers. There is a fair degree of agreement between the number of children desired for oneself and the number regarded as ideal for the average family. The average number of children born thus far to the women in the sample is 2.26. The average number expected is 2.82. Thus on average each woman expects .56 additional children. Or to put it more realistically, somewhere around 60 per cent of the women expect to have no more children since their actual and expected fertility is the same. Fecundity in this population appears to be normal. Thus a higher order of effectiveness in the use of birth control will be required to realize the family-size desires that are expressed. As we shall see later there has been a switch to more effective means of birth control—a fact which may be reflected in the lower estimated number of additional children. In addition it seems reasonable to anticipate that the level of voluntary sterilization will increase as simple procedures such as vasectomy and laparotomy become more popular. It seems inevitable that despite all this there will be some excess fertility although even with some lowering of family-size norms we would expect that the relative amount of unwanted fertility would be much less than in the recent past. We have this prognosis on the trend towards more effective contraception. Should abortion on demand become readily available the amount of unwanted fertility could be expected to reach unprecedented low levels. Part of any excess fertility will undoubtedly be taken care of through the elasticity of family-size desires—the rest representing failure both personal and social. Since this survey is limited to married couples we have no way of telling how well regulated the fertility of unmarried persons might be. Glancing once again south of our borders for some indication of what might obtain here, the likelihood is that the relatively high order of efficiency in fertility regulation achieved by married couples is attained by only a small fraction of the unmarried who are sexually active.[25] Thus any reflections on the amount of personal and social failure involved in fertility regulation in metropolitan Canada must bear in mind the limitation of our sample with respect to the civil status of the respondents.

Religious affiliation is very closely related to fertility. Catholics have higher actual and expected fertility than Protestants. However, the differences between Catholic and non-Catholic fertility seem to be smaller in our sample than those found in national surveys done in the United States.

There is a significant association between our measure of religiosity and actual and expected fertility both for Protestants and Catholics. Those who attend church more often have more children irrespective of their religious affiliation. For Catholics, however, one must attain approximately a weekly schedule of attendance before it makes any difference. With respect to fertility, to be a Catholic has little positive effect on fertility unless one is also a "good" Catholic in the sense of going regularly to Mass.

Educational attainment of the wife does not have as clear an inverse relation to fertility as has generally been observed in the past. Among the highly educated, especially among highly educated Catholics, fertility is above average. Income does not show any association with fertility.

Labour force participation has a significant relation not only to current fertility but to total expected fertility. The largest differentials among those so far examined are found for wife's labour force participation. Even when all other factors are controlled, labour force participation does not diminish in importance. This relationship is of course two edged—low fertility can promote labour force participation as well as the reverse. Early initiation into the labour force by

[25] Zelnik and Kantner, "Sexuality, Contraception, and Pregnancy Among Pre-Adult Females in the United States."

itself has relatively little effect on expected fertility except among those whose work exposure before the first birth exceeds ten years. This latter finding is consistent with the notion that to establish an alternative to domestic activity may have a depressing effect on ultimate fertility. It suggests however that this is not accomplished by a brief exposure to the labour force. Selectivity in terms of subfecundity would not seem to be an explanation in this instance since, to the extent that our data permitted, we controlled for fecundity.

Unlike the situation in the United States, nativity remains a crucial variable in explaining fertility differentials in Canada. Foreign-born women, especially from northwest Europe, prescribe a smaller family for the average Canadian family than is prescribed by a native-born Canadian and desire an even smaller family for themselves. Their actual and expected fertility is similarly below that of native-born women.

3

Timing and Spacing of Births

In Canada, much less is known about trends and differentials in the age at marriage and timing of births than about trends in levels of fertility. The Canadian Census collects data for married women on children ever born and publishes cumulative birth rates per 1,000 women in specified ages. However, as these cumulative birth rates are based on different cohorts they reveal nothing about childspacing within various cohorts. Nor can such information be derived from vital statistics data as birth certificates lack information about the timing of previous births.

Thus it was necessary to collect data on timing of births retrospectively. In our survey, detailed information was collected on childspacing and age at marriage. The importance of timing or childspacing is obvious for even if total completed family size does not vary among various cohorts of women the birth rate can vary as a result of variation in the timing of births. The investigation of timing of births may well be, as some students have suggested, more important than the study of the total number of births born to a woman in her lifetime.

In this chapter we shall be concerned with the following questions: At what age have women been marrying? Does a woman's socioeconomic background or labour force participation affect her spacing of children? What is the influence of family planning practices on childspacing? Before attempting to answer these questions, however, we shall examine the spacing patterns themselves as revealed in an

Table 22 Mean Age at Marriage and Mean Length of Birth Intervals by Age of Wife at Time of Survey

				Average No. of Months				Per Cent Having			
Age of Wife	*Number of Wives*	*Age at Marriage*	*Marriage Duration*	*Marriage to 1st*	*1st to 2nd*	*2nd to 3rd*	*3rd to 4th*	*1st*	*2nd*	*3rd*	*4th*
Less than 24	195	19.4	3.0	15	24	21	34	64	26	5	1
25–29	322	21.1	5.9	23	29	31	21	77	50	19	5
30–34	329	21.9	10.3	26	34	33	28	91	80	41	17
35–39	358	23.0	14.0	29	36	39	35	92	77	51	24
40 or more	426	23.3	19.2	33	40	49	46	92	79	46	24
All women	1630	22.0	11.7	27	35	39	37	85	66	36	16

analysis of the mean age at marriage and the mean length of birth intervals[1] by age of mother.

The figures in table 22 must be interpreted with caution, as mean age at marriage and mean birth intervals are a function of present age and marriage duration. Older women will tend to have a higher age at marriage and longer average birth intervals because they have greater opportunity to marry late or postpone births. In addition, our concern with only married women who have never been divorced can be expected to have a selective effect that would bias the data when they are classified by age. Ideally we would like to observe all women in a birth cohort throughout their entire reproductive period. However, as our sample consists of various cohorts at different stages of childbearing, age directly influences the various timing measures. As such, while the figures in table 22 give the pattern of childspacing within each group, they are not strictly comparable between age groups. We can, however, make certain comments about events that are not likely to show much change as age and marriage duration increase. For example, among women over 30 the percentage having a first child is the same in each age subclass suggesting that mean values relative to the early period of family formation have stabilized for each of these subgroups. Notice therefore that for these older women the mean age at marriage and the interval between marriage and first birth have been going down. This is a reminder of the advanced time schedules characteristic of the baby boom of the 1950s. Women who were 30 to 34 at the time of the survey were, on average, getting married and starting their families at the height of the baby boom. Their short initial birth interval of 26 months was in fact one of the factors in the boom. By way of contrast, women 40 and over were beginning their married lives in the immediate post-war years in the midst of a housing shortage, rationing, and a fair degree of uncertainty in the economic outlook. It is interesting that this group does not seem to have attempted to "catch up" on their birth schedule by shortening the second interval.

Socio-Economic Differences in Age at Marriage and the Timing of Births

For various socio-economic groups, the average age at marriage and

[1] Intervals are calculated by taking the difference between events in days and converting this difference back into months. An interval of 14 months would imply a range from 13.5 to 14.5 months.

the birth intervals are presented in table 23. The table also provides data on marriage duration and the percentage having different numbers of births. Since the sample contains women of different ages, these percentages, when multiplied successively, do not produce parity progression ratios. True parity progression ratios will be much higher. Also, as the higher intervals represent the experience of a small number of women, we should place less confidence in these intervals than in the first and second intervals.

Age at marriage is influenced only slightly by socio-economic factors other than the wife's education and her labour force status before marriage. Those who had some college education married on an average about two years later than those with less than three years of high school. Similarly, those who had a job before marriage had an average age at marriage of 22.3 while those not in the labour force married earlier at an average age of 20.7. However, about 87 per cent were in the labour force before marriage. There is no evidence that a career orientation has much effect on the average age at marriage. Length of employment after marriage appears to have no association with age at marriage. It would appear that once a woman reaches age 22 she has had time to gain work experience and an education. The important fact would seem to be that marriage and work, even that positively valued kind of work we call a career—are quite compatible. The critical decision is childbirth, not marriage.

There is an observable tendency for upper status women to have married somewhat later. This shows up in the distribution of average age at marriage by husband's income and his occupation at marriage and at present. Here again, however, the strong convergence around age 22 is an impressive fact. Age at marriage in contemporary Canada is not a variable with much demographic impact. The adaptation of demographic behaviour to social realities apparently comes largely in the choice of family-size goals and in the timing patterns followed subsequent to marriage in arriving at these goals. The timing of births may have a lot to do with the choice of goals. The means may determine the ends as much as the ends determine the means.

If the foregoing argument is valid we would expect to find difference by socio-economic status in the spacing of births. Only the first interval, the one between marriage and first birth, shows significant variation by socio-economic characteristics. Hardly any pattern is evident in the higher intervals.

Variation in the length of the first interval by socio-economic status is generally consistent with the idea that the higher the status the greater the tendency to postpone the first birth. There are some interesting exceptions to this however. College-educated women have a slightly shorter interval than wives who only went to high school. However, since proportionately fewer of the college women have had a first birth we might expect the length of the interval to change, most probably by becoming larger, as more embark on parenthood.

The relationship by husband's income is J shaped rather than linearly positive. Less than half of the lowest income group have progressed from marriage to parenthood. If the more fecund and less careful are selected for early motherhood the tendency would be for this J shape to become more pronounced as time passes. One is tempted to note the lack of any support in these figures for the common middle-class notion that early marriage and early childbearing are characteristic of low-income couples.

The most important variable seems to be the wife's labour force status before and after marriage. Women who worked before marriage not only married late but waited for a longer time before first birth. This is no doubt because proportionately more who worked before marriage worked after marriage. Period of work after marriage is highly correlated to first birth interval. However, interpretation of this relationship is hazardous as being childless is also conducive to being in the labour force.

Economic Consequences of Childspacing[2]

Thus far in this chapter we have been examining socio-economic variables for their effect on childspacing. In recent years since the publication by Freedman and Coombs[3] of their analysis of the relationship for a sample of Detroit women interest has developed in the possibility that the timing of births may itself influence economic status. The results of the few studies that have been made of this relationship have tended to confirm the relationship, especially with respect to the economic handicaps that seem to follow from a premarital pregnancy. The mechanism of action is not clear although it has been suggested that early involvement in childbearing diverts family resources, including time, away from activities that might promote economic advancement. This is perhaps the case especially

2 This section is based on analysis undertaken by Dr. Trinidad Osteria as part of her doctoral work at the Johns Hopkins University.

3 Freedman and Coombs, "Childspacing and Family Economic Position." Also Coombs, Freedman, Freedman, and Pratt, "Premarital Pregnancy and Status Before and After Marriage."

with the husband's education. Presser makes the argument that the timing of the first birth is critical with respect to the wife's economic role.[4] Domesticity tends to breed domesticity. Thus it seems plausible that a couple that enters on parenthood early may have less to put into the struggle to get ahead and, faced with high opportunity costs at a crucial time in their own period of economic take off, may become demoralized in addition.

To test this proposition requires that account be taken of other factors related to economic success and that there be control for the duration of marriage since both income and asset accumulation are time dependent. There is clear evidence in table 24 that premarital pregnancy is associated with below average current income after control for several factors that are known determinants of income. Premarital pregnancy was estimated as having occurred in all cases where the first child was born within six months of marriage. It would seem therefore that these data confirm the previous findings relative to the negative income effect of a premarital pregnancy.

To put this conclusion in perspective, however, it should be noted that the analysis is limited to women of the first four parities among whom only about 10 per cent had experienced a premarital pregnancy by the criterion here employed. It must also be noted that control over the social and economic condition at the outset of marriage while as good or better than in previous studies is less adequate than we would like. Premarital pregnancy was found to occur disproportionately among couples where the wife's or husband's father had only an elementary education. Thus though the procedures followed here are comparable and in some ways more adequate than those followed in previous tests of the relationship and although our results are similar in so far as the gross appearance of the relationship is concerned, there is reason to believe that a more complete apprehension of the couple's social and economic context in early marriage might seriously attenuate these results. With respect to the economic effects of childspacing; that is, the interval to first and subsequent births, we could find no consistent evidence of the relationship reported by others although admittedly the analysis is plagued by small numbers in some categories.

Going beyond husband's current income we examined to see whether the effects of childspacing would show up in other measures of economic advancement or economic position: measures such as change in income from marriage to the present, intergenerational

[4] Presser, "The Timing of First Births, Female Roles and Black Fertility."

Table 23 Mean Age at Marriage; Marriage Duration; Length of Birth Intervals; Percentage Having Specified Number of Births; Actual and Expected Births for Selected Characteristics

				Months between Births									
Characteristic	*No. of Wives*	*Age at Marriage*	*Years Married*	*Marriage to 1st*	*1st to 2nd*	*2nd to 3rd*	*3rd to 4th*	*Percentage Having 1st*	*2nd*	*3rd*	*4th*	*Actual Births*	*Expected Births*
Total	1632	22.0	11.7	27	35	38	37	85	66	37	17	2.25	2.82
Wife's Religion													
Protestant	976	22.0	11.9	30	34	38	40	83	66	35	16	2.14	2.69
Catholic	498	22.1	11.3	22	35	37	32	88	73	45	23	2.51	3.10
Jewish	62	22.1	13.0	33	40	41	34	87	74	34	13	2.19	2.82
Other	96	22.0	11.1	20	36	49	47	84	63	34	11	2.08	2.63
Wife's Education													
Less than 8 yrs.	363	21.7	13.2	23	39	44	38	92	76	44	19	2.67	2.99
High school 1–3	601	21.4	12.1	28	34	38	35	88	68	36	16	2.33	2.80
High school 4–5	476	22.6	11.3	30	34	39	39	81	60	31	15	2.01	2.67
College	190	23.6	9.0	27	31	35	36	76	61	32	14	1.89	2.89
Nativity of Wife													
Native born	956	21.9	11.6	28	34	36	38	83	67	38	19	2.27	2.89
Foreign born	673	22.3	11.9	25	36	41	37	88	69	36	15	2.22	2.75

Table 23 (Continued)

Characteristic	*No. of Wives*	*Age at Marriage*	*Years Married*	*Months between Births* Marriage to 1st	*1st to 2nd*	*2nd to 3rd*	*3rd to 4th*	*Percentage Having* 1st	*2nd*	*3rd*	*4th*	*Actual Births*	*Expected Births*
Wife's Labour Force Status before Marriage													
In labour force	1413	22.3	11.6	28	35	37	37	84	67	37	17	2.23	2.80
Not in labour force	219	20.7	12.5	20	37	44	37	92	76	43	20	2.44	2.87
Wife's Labour Force Status after Marriage													
6 months' work	813	21.7	11.3	14	31	38	39	31	26	41	21	2.30	2.96
7–12 months	283	22.3	11.4	19	34	34	34	96	76	12	20	2.60	2.06
13–18 months	98	22.6	10.5	24	35	39	*	91	73	40	17	2.25	2.87
19–24 months	100	22.9	12.1	35	38	36	*	95	78	34	12	2.35	2.63
25–36 months	109	22.3	12.2	40	35	38	*	95	64	27	11	2.02	2.50
37–48 months	59	22.7	12.3	49	36	*	*	88	61	29	12	1.93	2.47
49–60 months	46	22.7	13.3	62	41	*	*	83	52	13	*	1.70	2.04
61–84 months	60	22.2	13.8	72	43	*	*	93	63	18	02	1.68	2.08

More than 85 months	33	22.7	15.7	97	*	*	*	79	48	21	03	1.45	1.64
No response	31	21.6	12.5	25	*	*	*	65	55	39	16	2.00	2.71
Husband's Income													
$4000	112	22.3	10.6	28	31	39	*	46	36	34	16	2.03	3.04
$4000–$5999	417	21.8	11.0	22	37	36	35	84	66	37	17	2.27	2.87
$6000–$7999	395	21.9	11.3	26	35	36	36	85	62	32	17	2.12	2.77
$8000–$9999	228	21.8	11.7	31	33	43	38	85	68	38	15	2.15	2.76
$10000–$11999	180	22.5	12.3	31	36	37	34	89	75	40	16	2.28	2.59
$12000 or more	182	22.7	13.7	30	32	40	48	94	80	52	23	2.62	2.90
No Response	118	22.1	12.4	27	36	41	38	87	74	41	22	2.53	2.88
Husband's Occupation at Marriage													
Upper white collar	340	22.7	11.5	28	32	37	44	83	67	40	17	2.18	2.90
Lower white collar	429	21.8	11.3	31	35	38	38	85	65	37	17	2.13	2.63
Blue collar	825	21.8	12.4	25	37	40	34	87	70	38	18	2.35	2.82
Husband's Present Occupation													
Upper white collar	615	22.6	12.0	30	34	36	38	86	71	40	19	2.27	2.83
Lower white collar	284	22.0	10.9	28	34	39	39	81	60	33	12	2.00	2.63
Blue collar	717	21.7	11.9	24	36	40	36	87	70	39	18	2.35	2.88

**Average not given as it is based on number of cases below 25.*

Table 24 Husband's Current Income by Wife's Premarital Pregnancy Status and Current Parity

Current Parity and Premarital Pregnancy Status	*Mean Income* *Unadjusted*	*Adjusted**	*N*
Parity 1			
Premarital pregnancy	6612.50	7097.50	29
No premarital pregnancy	7719.50	8102.50	239
Parity 2			
Premarital pregnancy	7200.00	7837.50	45
No premarital pregnancy	8476.00	8842.50	377
Parity 3			
Premarital pregnancy	7580.00	7885.00	31
No premarital pregnancy	9014.50	9820.00	243
Parity 4			
Premarital pregnancy	6307.50	7535.00	13
No premarital pregnancy	9258.50	10430.00	126

**Adjusted for husband's education, religion, church attendance, and duration of marriage.*

occupation mobility, and relative income.[5] The results were essentially negative.

There is no clear explanation for the difference in behaviour of the Toronto couples and the Detroit couples. A comparison of the two samples reveals that in general the Detroit couples had somewhat lower income at each parity;[6] lower occupational status; proportionately more wives with only an elementary education; two to three times as much premarital pregnancy at each parity; and considerably different distribution by length of birth interval. For example, among parity one women, over half of the Detroit couples had their first birth within 12 months; for Toronto couples a little over one quarter did so. Large differences of this type are observable also at parities two and four. What this means is not obvious except that Detroit is a much different place from Toronto and that a relationship found in one place may not necessarily hold in the other. However, the generality of the income effect of childspacing is limited. The next step is not to rest with this but to attempt to discover the condition under which it does and does not operate.

[5] Income was classified as high–medium–low on the basis of its comparison with an expected income based on a regression between income and education, age, occupation, and place of birth.

[6] Comparisons were made only for parities 1, 2, and 4.

Distribution of Birth Intervals

The mean length of interval can be deceptive as the distribution of birth intervals is often very skewed. For first births, the mode is ten months and median 18 months, while the mean is 27 months. As many as 14 per cent of the first births occurred in the first eight months, suggesting pregnancy at the time of marriage. This percentage of pregnant brides is similar across the various socio-economic groups. There are relatively few illegitimate births, as opposed to premarital conceptions. First birth occurred before marriage only in 2 per cent of the cases.

Some idea of skewness in the distribution of birth intervals by different orders can be inferred from table 25. Comparison of means and medians for higher order birth intervals seems to indicate that skewness is less in these cases than among first order births.

The distribution of first birth intervals varies widely by wife's religion and education (table 26). Catholics have their first births much earlier than other religious groups. More than two-thirds of Catholic wives had their first child within two years of marriage as compared to 56 per cent of Protestants.

Table 25 Mode, Median, and Mean of Different Birth Intervals

Interval in Months	*Marriage to First*	*First to Second*	*Second to Third*	*Third to Fourth*
Number of wives	1393	1110	612	279
Mode	10	15	*	*
Median	18	28	32	31
Mean	27	35	38	37

No clear mode.

An examination of the shape of the birth interval distributions therefore reveals something of the heterogeneity within groups with respect to timing. Although the mean length of the first interval for Protestants is 30 months, half had their first child within 22 months of marriage. Another way of putting this is to say that while on average Protestants had their first child after two and a half years of marriage, the proportion who waited three or more years (30 per cent) is greater than the proportion who had a birth in the first year of marriage (27 per cent). Among Catholics, on the other hand, the proportion who waited three or more years (16 per cent) is less than

Table 26 Percentage Distribution of Time between Marriage and First Birth, for Wives by Religion and Education

Charac-teristic	*Number of Wives*	*Total*	*Years between Marriage and First Birth* Under 1 Year	1–1.99 years	2–2.99 years	3–4.99 years	5–6.99 years	7 or more
Total	1393*	100	30	32	14	14	6	4
Wife's Religion								
Protestant	812	100	27	29	14	17	8	5
Catholic	440	100	36	34	14	10	4	2
Other	141	100	28	38	11	13	6	4
Wife's Education								
Less than 8 yrs.	333	100	33	36	13	12	5	2
High school 1–3 yrs.	529	100	31	32	12	14	6	5
High school 4–5 yrs.	387	100	26	30	16	15	7	6
College	144	100	32	26	18	13	8	3

**33 wives who had a first birth before marriage are not included.*

half the proportion who had a birth in the first year of marriage (36 per cent). If we consider that most of those who delivered in the first 23 months of married life became pregnant within 14 months after marriage and further that this represents 70 per cent of the Catholics, a mean monthly fecundability of about .08 is implied.[7] A mean monthly fecundability of .08 for women of zero parity is substantially lower (by half or more) than would be expected if no contraception were being employed.[8] We have no knowledge of the nature of contraceptive practices by Catholic women during this first interval, whether it consisted of widespread but somewhat ineffective use, some mixture of effective use and non-use, or some other com-

[7] If p is mean monthly fecundability, the proportion pregnant by the end of n months is given by the formula: Proportion pregnant $= p+pq+pq^2+pq^3+\cdots+pq^{n-1} = 1-q^n$ where $q = 1-p$. Solving $.7 = 1-q^{14}$ yields a value for $q = .918$ or $p = .082$.

[8] Tietze, "Probability of Pregnancy Resulting From a Single Unprotected Coitus." Potter, "Some Physical Correlates of Fertility Control in the United States."

bination. In the absence of contraception, assuming a mean monthly fecundability of .18, more than twice the observed value, 70 per cent of the newly married would have been pregnant in six months rather than in 14. Thus though Catholic women were not distinguished as a group by highly effective contraception in the period from marriage to their first birth, they nevertheless delayed their first pregnancy to a significant degree. The implied mean monthly fecundability for Protestants is about half that estimated from these data for Catholics. Thus it would require about 26 months—one year more than for Catholics—for 70 per cent of the newly-married Protestants to become pregnant. These are very large differences which, as we shall see later, the contraceptive revolution of recent years will no doubt diminish greatly.

Analysis of Childspacing Using Closed and Open Intervals

Our analysis till now has been based on "closed" birth intervals; in other words to intervals which ended in a birth. "Open" intervals, or the interval since the birth of the last child to the time of the survey did not enter into the calculations. Thus the first birth interval of 27 months from marriage to first birth is based on 1,393 women who had a first birth by the time of the survey. However, many of the women who had not had a first birth by the time of the survey are likely to have it later. As the sample is composed of various age cohorts of women, many of them having different durations of exposure still left for future fertility in their reproductive period, their fertility is an incomplete picture of their reproductive performance. This truncation of the reproductive period poses problems of measurement in childspacing measures. Period of observation has a direct effect both on closed and open intervals, that is, on the interval between successive births and the interval since the most recent birth. The longer the period of observation, the longer the interval is likely to be. A finite duration of observation will also have a tendency to decrease intervals of higher parity. The implications of truncation on spacing have been examined recently but no proper solution has been found because of the complex nature of the interrelationships involved.[9]

[9] Potter, "Birth Intervals: Structure and Change." Srinivasan, "Findings and Implications of a Correlation Analysis of the Closed and Open Birth Intervals." Sheps, *et al.*, "Birth Intervals: Artifact and Reality," pp. 857-68. Sheps, *et al.*, "Truncation Effects in Birth Interval Data."

By combining both closed and open intervals and using life table techniques, we can construct probabilities of births and birth delays as well as other childspacing measures, which also include the past experiences of women lost to follow-up.[10] Probabilities of births and birth delays at various durations are presented in table 27. The probability of a woman giving birth to a child in the first two years of marriage is .57. The fairly high probability of .178 for the first nine months indicates a substantial proportion pregnant at the time of marriage. 4.6 per cent of the women are likely to remain childless even after a long period of exposure to pregnancy. Comparison with first interval reveals that second births are delayed longer than first births, in part because of the inclusion of illegitimate conceptions in the first interval. Cumulative probability of having a birth reaches .57 only after three years while in the case of first birth it was reached in two years.

Table 27 Cumulative Probabilities of Birth and Birth Delays for the First and Second Births

	First Birth		*Second Birth*	
Duration in Months	*Cumulative Probability of Birth since Marriage*	*Cumulative Probability of Birth Delay*	*Cumulative Probability of Birth since First Birth*	*Cumulative Probability of Birth Delay*
1–9	.178	.822	.003	.997
10–12	.302	.698	.041	.959
13–24	.571	.429	.354	.646
25–36	.700	.300	.575	.425
37–48	.787	.213	.702	.298
49–60	.830	.170	.787	.213
61–72	.868	.132	.832	.168
73–84	.897	.103	.859	.141
85–120	.934	.066	.894	.106
121–204	.954	.046	.923	.077
205+	.954	.046	.923	.077

A measure of interest in fertility research is the proportion of women who pass from one parity to the next. In a cross-section

[10] See Appendix C for a detailed discussion and analysis of the life-table study of childspacing.

sample such as ours it is not possible to calculate the "parity progression ratios" for all the women as they are at various stages of their reproductive career. Only for women over 40 years of age can the parity distribution at the time of the survey be assumed to be reasonably close to the completed parity distribution. Often sample size in this group is small and represents the experience of one particular cohort only. However, the cumulative probabilities in table 27 provide crude approximations to these parity progression ratios. Cumulative probabilities reach a constant value after a long period. If we assume that births are not likely to take place after such a long period as is the case with the sample women, we can treat these as the proportions who are likely to go on to the next parity. The parity progression ratios so computed are given below.

Parity Progression Ratios

1.	(Marriage to first)	.954
2.	(First to second)	.927
3.	(Second to third)	.702
4.	(Third to fourth)	.636
5.	(Fourth to fifth)	.572
6.	(Fifth to sixth)	.515

It should be emphasized that these are hypothetical measures combining the experience of all the cohorts of women in the sample. The implied final distribution compared to the actual parity distribution is shown in table 28.

The total fertility rate computed on the basis of PPR's is approximately 3.254, while the mean current fertility of the sample was 2.26. The difference may be interpreted as the future expected fertility among the sample women on the basis of their past fertility performance alone; in other words, if a woman were to follow the reproductive pathway of the average woman in this sample she would have 3.25 births by the time she was done. In the survey, the women were asked how many additional children they expect to have. The mean total expected family size thus constructed was only 2.82. Whether the actual completed family size will be this value will be a function of the couple's ability to achieve the exact additional number they want. The difference between the total fertility rate derived from PPRs and the total expected births may possibly be seen as indicative of a decline in the family-size norms in our sample women. It could also indicate the extent to which the best laid plans may go awry.

Table 28 Percentage Distribution of Sample Women by Number of Births at the Time of the Survey and by End of Reproductive Period as Implied by Parity Progression Ratios

Number of Children	*At Survey Date*	*At End of Reproductive Period as Implied by PPRs*
0	12.6	4.6
1	18.4	7.0
2	31.2	26.3
3	20.3	22.6
4	10.2	16.9
5	4.2	11.0
6+	3.1	11.6

Measures of Childspacing

Closed and open intervals are a function of length of the observation period. This effect was noticed earlier in the discussion of table 22. The length of the closed interval increases with the age of the woman. Thus, the commonly used measures of mean interval for the whole sample underestimate the interval that would have obtained had the women been observed for the entire reproductive period. Moreover, as the means are a function of the distribution by age, comparisons of means between surveys will be invalid to the extent that these are age distribution differences. Life-table techniques provide a way of adjusting these intervals for incomplete periods of observation.

The effect of the life-table approach to the calculation of closed intervals can be observed in table 29.

While the life-table means are higher for all interval orders, they are far from uniform. Differences are larger for middle parities and smaller for other parities. Differences will depend on the shape of closed and open interval distributions, and on the truncation effect for different parities. Even the life-table means have a truncation effect for higher parities as can be seen from the declining values for means.

A combined study of closed and open intervals through life-table techniques provides one way of computing synthetic measures. It should be realized that they are constructs from the combined experience and do not refer to any particular cohort of women. The approach also provides a method for adjusting interval data for women lost to observation. The truncation effect still persists in life-table means, but they at least adjust for varying periods of exposure of sample women during their reproductive periods.

Summary

Comparisons among older cohorts (those over 30) seem to indicate a decline in age at marriage. Age at marriage shows some positive association with wife's education and there is a tendency for wives who worked before marriage to marry later. Those who belong to the upper social class as indicated by income and occupation of the husband marry somewhat later, a relationship which is doubtless confounded with the education of the wife. In no case is the mean difference as much as two years.

Table 29 Mean Length of Closed Intervals: Direct and Life-Table Calculation

	Sample $\bar{x}^i$		*Life Table $\bar{x}^i$*	
Interval Order	*Number of Women*	*Interval in Months*	*Base Number of Women Observed*	*Interval in Months*
1 (marriage to first)	1393	27.06	1599	30.07
2	1110	34.93	1393	38.64
3	603	38.85	1110	45.94
4	279	37.20	603	49.52
5	113	34.16	279	42.34
6	45	30.73	113	33.12

Variations of half a year or more in childspacing are to be observed, at least for the interval from marriage to first birth, by religion, education, wife's labour force status, and husband's occupation. These differences are generally attenuated at higher birth orders. Differences greater than one year are exceptional except in the case of the wife's work experience after marriage. In demographic terms differences in the length of the first and subsequent birth intervals are of consequence only if the total number of births is affected and if the average age at which women have their babies shifts in an upward or downward direction. Important also in this connection is the starting point: the age at marriage. For example, an average Protestant and an average Catholic woman, both of whom married at age 22 and who were to have four children each, would arrive at their fourth birth within about a year and a half of each other if they followed an average pattern of birth intervals. Of much greater demographic impact are the differences in the proportions who progress from one parity to the next. However, the significance of a six to eight month difference in a birth interval, especially the first one during which a newly formed family is marshalling its resources and energies, could well be of tremendous importance. This aspect of the process of family building and its consequences has not been studied to our knowledge.

An examination of the effect of spacing patterns on income confirms previous findings with respect to premarital pregnancy which tends to have a negative effect upon husband's income in later years. There is reason to believe, however, that tighter analysis might weaken the relationship which in any case currently involves only a small percentage of couples.

A life-table analysis reveals interesting patterns which are lost if only mean intervals are considered. A probability distribution of births is a function of many factors, such as use of family planning, accidental pregnancies, and extent of sub-fecundity. It is interesting to observe that these factors tend to produce a random distribution of birth probabilities. Life-table analysis also provides a way of calculating parity progression ratios and mean intervals, even though they are based on different cohorts of women. It should be emphasized that there may be families of decrement tables appropriate for various types of population having a broad utility such as has been experienced with model life tables for mortality. Further investigation of attrition patterns by childbirth for specified populations is recommended.

4

Family Limitation

In this chapter we are concerned with the attitudes of wives towards the use of contraception and the extent of the use of contraception to voluntarily limit or plan families. The specific methods used will also be investigated. A more detailed analysis of oral contraception use will be the topic of Chapter 5.

We mean by contraception any method used with the intention of preventing a conception. It includes oral pills, intra-uterine devices, mechanical and chemical methods, rhythm, douche, abstinence, and coitus interruptus or withdrawal.

Attitudes towards Family Limitation

The widespread acceptance of contraception is evident in the fact that 86 per cent approved of contraception without any qualifications and another seven per cent approved with some qualifications.

This finding is based on responses to the question: "Many couples use contraceptives to limit the size of their family or to have their children when they want them. We would like to hear some of your views on this subject. First, in general do you approve of married couples doing something to plan their families? [Probe]"

Variations in degree of approval were more closely associated with religion than with any other characteristic. Among Protestants 96 per cent approved of birth control as compared to 66 per cent among

Catholics (table 30). Catholics were the only group where there was a significant percentage either not approving family limitation or attaching qualifications to their approval. Because of the small number who disapprove of birth control, no further analysis is made within religious groups by factors such as education and religiosity which might further clarify the relationship.

Use of Contraception

A large majority of women in our sample are using or have used some form of contraception. We have defined a user as one who has employed any of the methods listed above for the purpose of preventing a pregnancy. We deal with abortion in Chapter 6. Data on contraceptive use were collected by asking whether contraception was ever used, whether it is being used now, how extensively and how effectively it has been used, and what methods have been used. Special attention is paid to the use of oral contraception because of the rapidly growing importance of this method. We devote the whole of Chapter 5 to the analysis of oral contraceptive use. Here we are concerned with the extent of use, its socio-economic correlates, and the distribution of users by contraceptive methods.

Table 30 Percentage Distribution of Wife's Attitude towards Family Planning by Religion of Wife

		Attitudes towards Family Planning				
Religion of Wife	*Number of Wives*	*Approval*	*Qualified**	*Disapproval*	*Non-response*	*Total*
Protestant	976	96	1	3	—	100
Catholic	498	66	15	16	3	100
Jewish	62	94	6	0	—	100
Others	96	83	8	8	1	100
Total	1632	86	6	7	1	100

**Qualified responses include answers such as "all right for others," "up to the individual," etc.*

Among the sample couples, 83 per cent had used contraception at some time. Even among the 12 per cent who reported sterility at the time of the survey, two-thirds had used contraception earlier.

At the time of the survey, 63 per cent of all women were using some form of contraception (table 31). Among fecund women, this percentage is 71 per cent and among those actually exposed to the risk of pregnancy (fecund women excluding those pregnant at the time of the survey) the percentage of users is 75 per cent. Of the 25 per cent of fecund women not using contraception more than half wished to become pregnant. Thus the amount of unprotected exposure among fecund women who did not want to become pregnant was just under 13 per cent.[1]

Demographic Correlates of Family Limitation

Except for women 40 or over who are also likely to be longest married, contraceptive use does not vary much by age. About two-thirds of all women in the different age categories currently use some form of contraception. Age differences remain insignificant even if we limit ourselves to fecund women or women exposed to risk (table 32). Any variations in current use by age among women under 40 is attributable to the differential prevalence of pregnancy.

Table 31 Percentage of Women Using Contraception by Risk Status

Use of Contraception	*All Women*	*Fecund Women*	*Fecund Women Excluding Those Pregnant*	*Fecund Women, Excluding Pregnant, Not Wanting Another Child*
Total	1,632	1,391	1,303	644
Ever used contraception	83	86	86	86
Currently using contraception	63	71	75	79

Marriage duration makes little difference in the percentage who have ever used contraception except for those married 21 years or more among whom nearly one in four have never used. The highest level of current use is among those women exposed to risk in the two

[1] 75 per cent using and presumed not to want pregnancy. 11 per cent not using and presumed not to want pregnancy. Unprotected exposure = 11/(75+11) = .13.

years immediately following marriage, indicating a concern with spacing in the early years of marriage. Conversely, current contraceptive use among women at risk is relatively low two to five years after marriage, a period when a considerable proportion of couples have their first and second children.

Current use among zero and one parity women is somewhat lower not only because many of them are trying to conceive but also due to the greater prevalence of sterility among this low fertility group. However, among women of these parities who are exposed to risk, use is comparable to the levels found among higher parity women.

The similarity among various age, parity, and duration categories in the extent of use seems to indicate that contraception is being used not only to limit family size, but to achieve a desired spacing. Unfortunately, we did not collect detailed data on contraceptive use history except in the case of oral contraception and therefore cannot investigate use at various stages of the reproductive career. There is a fairly high level of nonuse among older women, those married for a long time, and those who have five or more children even though only ten per cent of these women want more children.

Socio-Economic Correlates of Family Limitation

The influence of religious doctrine on the use of methods for limiting family size is evident when we look at Protestant–Catholic use patterns. Among Protestants, 69 per cent of all women were using some method at the time of the survey, this percentage increasing to 82 per cent among women exposed to risk. Among Catholics, however, the extent of use was lower at 51 per cent for all women and 61 per cent for women exposed to risk. "Ever use" is higher than current use for all religious groups but the relative rankings among fecund women or women exposed to risk remain the same. Only nine per cent of Protestant wives have never used contraception whereas more than 30 per cent of the comparable group of Catholic women have never used any method of birth control. The lesser current use among Jews overall is largely a matter of their relatively low fecundity. Current use among Jewish women rises from 55 to 70 per cent when infecund women are excluded.

An analysis of contraceptive use by wife's education reveals a distinct threshhold at the division between elementary and secondary education. Among women whose education ended below the ninth grade, only 43 per cent were currently using contraception in contrast

Table 32 Percentage of Current Users or Ever Users of Contraception by Age, Marriage Duration, and Parity of Women

	All Women			*Fecund Women*			*Women Exposed to Risk**		
Characteristic	*Number*	*Presently Using*	*Ever Used*	*Number*	*Presently Using*	*Ever Used*	*Number*	*Presently Using*	*Ever Used*
Total	1632	63	83	1391	71	86	1303	75	86
Age of Wife									
Less than 25	157	67	86	156	67	86	138	76	87
25–29	325	66	87	307	67	91	263	78	91
30–34	322	69	85	294	72	85	280	76	87
35–39	366	65	85	294	77	88	285	78	88
40 or more	462	53	74	340	69	81	337	69	81
Marriage Duration									
2 yrs. or less	156	68	84	150	70	86	130	81	89
2–5 yrs.	192	59	87	178	62	89	150	73	89
6–10 yrs.	400	68	85	368	71	86	343	76	87
11–15 yrs.	380	64	83	318	74	85	307	76	86
16–20 yrs.	318	64	82	254	76	85	250	77	86
21 or more	186	45	74	123	63	80	123	63	81
Number of Children									
0	206	46	74	151	60	85	129	71	88
1	300	52	79	258	58	82	223	67	83
2	509	71	85	466	76	87	449	78	87
3	332	66	85	277	76	86	268	77	86
4	166	73	88	148	80	89	145	81	90
5 or more	119	57	82	91	69	81	89	71	83

**Excluding currently pregnant.*

Table 33 Percentage of Current Users or Ever Users of Contraception by Selected Socio-Economic Characteristics

	All Women			*Fecund Women*			*Women Exposed to Risk*		
Characteristic	*Number*	*Presently Using*	*Ever Used*	*Number*	*Presently Using*	*Ever Used*	*Number*	*Presently Using*	*Ever Used*
Total	1632	63	83	1391	71	86	1303	75	86
Religion of Wife									
Protestant	976	69	91	838	78	94	788	82	94
Catholic	498	51	67	425	57	71	396	61	72
Jewish	62	55	87	47	70	91	42	79	95
Other	96	61	76	81	69	77	77	73	78
Education of Wife									
8th grade or less	363	43	59	308	49	61	289	52	63
9–11 grades	603	70	89	514	76	92	487	80	93
12–13 grades	476	67	89	401	76	92	372	82	92
College	190	73	94	168	79	95	155	85	95
Nativity of Wife									
Native born	958	68	90	804	77	94	752	83	94
Foreign born	674	54	72	587	62	75	551	65	75
Occupation of Husband									
Upper white collar	616	66	89	515	76	93	480	81	93
Lower white collar	284	65	87	238	76	91	223	81	92
Blue collar	718	59	75	624	65	78	588	69	79

to two-thirds or more of more highly educated women. Even among women at risk who had only an elementary education, only about half were using contraception as opposed to 80 per cent or more of the more educated groups. Since a disproportionate number of wives in the lowest education group were also Catholics, the low level of use is to some extent probably a joint effect of education and religion. Beyond eight years of education, there is a slight but discernible tendency for those with most education to display the highest levels of use. Under more refined analysis which would take account of age at marriage and marital duration the differences, especially for college women, might be somewhat greater, since as we saw in Chapter 3, college women married later, and have been married a shorter time. We would therefore expect more of them to have suspended contraception in order to conceive. There is, however, not much room for improvement since among college women exposed to risk 85 per cent are current users. With some allowance for known infecundity and planned pregnancy, only a marginal increase in the level of current use could be expected.

Consistent with the pattern for education, use among wives whose husbands are in blue-collar occupations is lower than among those whose husbands are in white-collar occupations. Differences within white-collar occupations are negligible.

Current and past contraceptive use is lower among the foreign born than among native-born women. Although the largest single category of foreign-born women are Western European Protestants, Catholics nevertheless comprise a greater proportion of the foreign born than of the native born. Thus the differences in contraceptive practice between the two groups are in the expected direction. Despite this, however, the fertility of foreign-born women is below that of native-born women. Age and marital duration distributions are similar for these two groups and in fact, control for these two factors somewhat increases the spread in fertility rates. Again there are differences within the foreign-born group with Western European Protestants displaying substantially lower actual, expected, or desired fertility than any other nativity group. The apparent paradox of less contraception and lower fertility exhibited by the foreign born thus appears to be partly compositional: the large proportion of Catholics among the foreign born pulls down the level of contraceptive use of the group overall; the use of contraception by other foreign-born women resembles that of native-born women but since the latter have very high levels of current and past use, there is little opportunity to better this performance. With respect to fertility it is the low fertility of foreign-born women from Western Europe, and to a lesser extent those from Eastern Europe, who are responsible for the below average achieved fertility of the group. These two groups together account for 63 per cent of all the foreign born. It is not surprising that the overall fertility of foreign-born women should be below that of Canadian-born women with so many originating from areas of Europe with some of the lowest fertility rates in the world. Some of these are also areas which in recent years have been characterized by a high prevalence of abortion. We do not know how many of the women in our sample have used abortion as a method of birth control but to the extent this is more true of the foreign born than of the native born this would help further to reconcile the picture of below average contraception and below average fertility which they present as a group. Other factors may also be involved, such as differences in the consistency and effectiveness of contraceptive use.[2] We do not have the data required to dispose finally of these perplexities. It is clear that to do so would entail detailed and separate analyses of different regional and religious subcategories among the foreign born.

Methods of Family Limitation Used

No previous data are available in Canada for use in investigating changes in the distribution of methods used for preventing conception. But when we compare use patterns among Toronto couples with earlier U.S. studies, we find the pattern of use is very different. While it is true that the samples are not strictly comparable as our sample is based only on a large metropolitan area, to a large extent this difference is due to the rapid adoption of oral contraception during the sixties, a trend which is more fully reflected in our data than in earlier studies.

The most common method is oral contraception among all the religious groups. Fifty per cent of all users among Protestants use oral contraception (table 34). Even among the Catholics, 43 per cent use orals. For the Protestants the next most popular method is the condom at 19.8 per cent. Use of the condom among Catholics is also significant at 15.1 per cent. The diaphragm while still an important method among Protestants and Jews is of minor importance among Catholics.

[2] It is possible, although we find little difference in de jure marital duration, that there could be de facto differences associated with disruptions related to emigration. These are thought to be minimal.

Table 34 Percentage Distribution of Current Users of Specified Methods of Contraception by Wife's Religion

Method	*Total*	*Protestant*	*Catholic*	*Jewish*	*Other*
Number of Users	1022	677	252	34	59
Oral pills	47.8	50.1	42.9	47.1	42.4
Condoms	18.5	19.8	15.1	17.7	18.6
Diaphragms	10.5	14.0	2.0	11.8	5.1
Rhythm	10.0	6.2	21.4	2.9	8.5
Withdrawal	9.8	7.2	13.9	8.8	22.0
I.U.D.'s	3.4	3.1	2.4	14.7	5.1
Jelly, cream, foam, and suppositories	3.7	4.3	1.6		8.5
Others (douching, abstinence, etc.)	3.9	2.1	8.0		8.5
Total percentage*	107.6	106.8	107.3	103.0	118.7

**Total exceeds 100.0 because of multiple use in some cases.*

Catholics rely to a greater extent than do Protestants on "natural" methods such as rhythm and withdrawal. As we shall see in the next chapter the advent of oral contraception has greatly reduced Catholic reliance on rhythm and withdrawal since over half of current oral users formerly used these methods. Nevertheless, the difference remains high with 21 per cent among Catholics compared with 6 per cent among Protestants reporting current use of rhythm or withdrawal. The extent of use of the rhythm method among Catholics in our sample is much less than is reported in earlier U.S. studies. Evidently this is a function of the increasing adoption of oral contraception among Catholics.[3] The relatively high prevalence of I.U.D. use among Jewish women is interesting but involves only a few women and is therefore of uncertain reliability.

[3] National fertility studies in the United States showed current rhythm use of 47 per cent in 1955, 45 per cent in 1960, and 34 per cent in 1965, among white Catholic users. Use of rhythm among Catholics in our sample prior to the widespread switch to orals appears to have been of a magnitude similar to that reported in the United States. Though we cannot provide a strictly comparable figure, the sum of those currently using rhythm plus those currently using orals whose last previous method was rhythm amounts to 35 per cent of current Catholic users.

In the rest of this chapter data on contraceptive use have been regrouped to take into account multiple use among some women. Almost half of all women using contraception are using oral pills only (table 35). Among Protestant users 83 per cent were either on pills, or such relatively effective methods as condoms, diaphragms, and intrauterine devices. Among Catholics, only 59 per cent were on these methods and 30 per cent were on such relatively ineffective methods as rhythm and withdrawal. This in conjunction with the lower overall prevalence of use among Catholics helps to explain, at least as regards means, the previously observed differences in Catholic fertility relative to other religious groups.

Table 35 Percentage Currently Using Specified Types of Contraception, by Wife's Religion

Type of Contraception	*Total*	*Protes-tant*	*Catholic*	*Others*
All Couples	1632	976	498	158
Total Per Cent	100	100	100	100
Non-Users	37	31	49	41
Users	63	69	51	59
Oral pills only	29	34	21	25
Appliance methods only	16	21	7	12
Rhythm only	4	2	9	2
Withdrawal only	5	4	6	7
I.U.D.'s only	2	2	1	5
Combinations of rhythm, withdrawal, and appliance	1	1	1	4
All others (douche, chemical methods, abstinence)	5	5	5	4
Users of Contraception	1022	677	252	93
Total Per Cent	100	100	100	100
Oral pills only	47	50	42	42
Appliance methods only	25	30	15	10
Rhythm only	7	3	19	3
Withdrawal only	8	5	11	12
I.U.D.'s only	3	3	2	9
Combinations of rhythm, withdrawal, and appliance	2	2	2	6
All others (douche, chemical methods, abstinence)	8	7	9	8

Interfaith marriages being somewhat uncommon, the differences in method preference observed by the wife's religion are essentially unchanged when both the wife's and husband's religious affiliation are considered (table 36). Because of small numbers, the findings for categories other than those in which husband and wife are either both Protestant or both Catholic must be interpreted with caution. Perhaps the most interesting effect of a mixed marriage in which only one partner is Catholic is the increase in the level of current use from less than 50 per cent for an unmixed Catholic marriage to around 67 per cent when either the wife or the husband is Protestant. Oral use also shows an increase under these conditions, especially when the non-Catholic is the wife.

If wife and husband are of different religious backgrounds, the wife's religion seems to be more influential than the husband's in the choice of the method. In those cases where the wife was Catholic and the husband Protestant, 17 per cent used rhythm only, while in the reverse situation sole users of rhythm were only four per cent. Consistently, use of orals was higher where the wife was Protestant than where her husband was Protestant. This would seem to indicate the dominance of the wife in family-planning decisions.

No clear pattern is observable in the use of contraception and church attendance. Among Catholics, oral pill use is noticeably higher among those who never go to church. However, among those who attend church sometimes there is an inexplicable upturn in the use of orals among those who attend most faithfully. Only in the case of rhythm can we observe a systematic increase in use with church attendance, both for Protestants and Catholics. Use of other methods appears to be uninfluenced by religious practice.

We observed in Chapter 2 that religiosity is positively related to actual and expected fertility. To some extent this may be explained by greater use among those who do not attend church often and a tendency for them also to show somewhat greater partiality towards oral contraception. Given the non-linearity of the relationship involving extent of use and type of method this cannot be more than a partial explanation of the differences in fertility. There are of course variations in effectiveness among users of the same method which we have not measured but which could be involved in the relationship. Moreover, current use is a less relevant measure in this connection than a measure such as ever use or intended use or some combination that would capture use over time.

Table 36 Percentage of Users Adopting Specified Types of Contraception by Couple's Religion

Type of Contraception	*Total*	*Both Protestant*	*Both Catholic*	*Both Jewish*	*Wife Protestant Husband Catholic*	*Wife Catholic Husband Protestant*	*Other*
Number of Couples	1632	921	437	60	44	54	116
Number of Users	1022	643	210	34	28	36	71
Percentage of Users	63	70	48	57	64	67	61
Percentage Total	100	100	100	100	100	100	100
Oral pills only	47	49	40	47	61	50	38
Appliance methods only	25	31	15	29	18	11	17
Rhythm only	7	3	20	0	4	17	4
Withdrawal only	8	6	11	6	4	14	14
All other and combinations	13	11	14	18	13	8	27

Demographic Correlates of Contraceptive Use Patterns

The wife's age is found to be significantly related to the type of contraception a couple adopts (table 38). Younger wives are predominantly oral pill users. Among women under 25, 68 per cent of all users are using oral contraception, the use being as high as 65 per cent even among young Catholic women. The extent of oral use decreases consistently with increase in the age of the wife. Only about one-third of women 40 and over are using the pill. As the oral pill is a recent method, many of the older women would have had to switch from methods to which they had become accustomed and found satisfactory. Also, being older they might be reluctant to adopt orals because of reported health hazards or because of a generally conservative attitude towards innovation either on their part or that of their physician. Some of these aspects of adoption will be analysed in greater detail in the next chapter. A crucial question concerning oral users, especially the younger women, is whether they will remain loyal to the method in the years to come. An analysis of continuation rates in the next chapter discloses a substantial degree of discontinuation for reasons other than to become pregnant.

Use of appliance methods, namely the condom and the diaphragm, is consistently higher among the older cohorts, and much more pronounced among Protestants than Catholics. These women started their reproductive life in the 1950s when the appliance methods were the most popular and dependable among the methods then available. The method currently used cannot of course be taken as an indication of the method of choice at an earlier age, but there is no doubt a degree of brand loyalty to be found here as in other areas of consumption. However, switching undoubtedly occurred in numerous cases.

Women currently using rhythm as the only method show practically no variation by age among Protestants, the level of use being a low three per cent. It is possible that some Protestant couples avoid coitus at what they regard as the dangerous time of the month but yet do not regard themselves as users of the "rhythm method" which they may associate with more elaborate measurement of cycle variability and temperature rather than mere calendar watching. One study with which we are familiar found a small percentage of women—young women under 20 in this case—reporting use of the "rhythm method" but at the same time a substantial proportion who failed to use birth control on their last sexual encounter, explained it by saying that "it was not the time of the month when I could get pregnant."

Table 37 Percentage Currently Using Specified Types of Contraception for All Couples and Users by Frequency of Wife's Church Attendance

Type	*Total*	*Never*	*Twice a Month or Less*	*Three or Four Times a Month*	*Five or More Times a Month*
			ALL COUPLES		
Number of Couples	1632	553	486	397	196
Per Cent Total	100	100	100	100	100
Non-Users	37	33	38	43	38
Users	63	67	62	57	62
Oral pills only	29	38	28	21	28
Appliance methods only	16	17	17	14	14
Rhythm only	4	1	3	8	10
Withdrawal only	5	3	6	5	4
I.U.D. only	2	2	1	2	2
Combinations of rhythm, withdrawal, and appliance	1	2	2	2	0
All others (douche, chemical methods, and abstinence	5	4	5	5	4
			PROTESTANT USERS		
Total Couples	961	400	306	172	83
Number of Users	672	276	217	115	64

Percentage of Users	70	69	71	67	77
Total Percentage of Users	100	100	100	100	100
Oral pills only	49	56	48	41	44
Appliance methods only	30	27	31	35	31
Rhythm only	4	1	3	6	11
Withdrawal only	5	5	7	3	6
I.U.D. only	3	3	2	3	3
Combinations of rhythm, withdrawal, and appliance	2	2	1	3	0
Others	7	6	8	9	5
			CATHOLIC USERS		
Total Couples	484	70	121	192	101
Number of Users	244	46	50	95	53
Percentage of Users	50	66	42	49	53
Total Percentage of Users	100	100	100	100	100
Oral pills only	42	63	32	34	49
Appliance methods only	15	15	22	13	11
Rhythm only	18	7	10	25	24
Withdrawal only	12	11	18	13	4
I.U.D. only	3	2	0	3	4
Combinations of rhythm, withdrawal, and appliance	1	0	4	1	0
Others	9	2	14	11	8

Table 38 Percentage Currently Using Specified Types of Contraception by Age of Wife and Religion

Type of Contraception	*Total*	*18–24*	*25–29*	*30–34*	*35–39*	*40 or older*
			TOTAL			
Number of users	1022	105	214	221	238	244
Percentage of users	100	100	100	100	100	100
Oral pills only	47	68	58	50	38	34
Appliance method only	25	11	19	22	29	36
Rhythm only	7	4	5	7	8	10
Withdrawal only	8	7	7	7	8	9
All others and combinations	13	10	11	14	17	11
			PROTESTANTS			
Number of users	677	64	137	140	158	178
Percentage of users	100	100	100	100	100	100
Oral pills only	50	75	60	54	40	38
Appliance method only	30	11	22	26	36	42
Rhythm only	3	0	4	2	4	5
Withdrawal only	5	5	5	5	6	6
All others and combinations	12	9	9	13	14	9
			CATHOLICS			
Number of users	252	28	58	60	56	50
Percentage of users	100	100	100	100	100	100
Oral pills only	42	65	53	42	34	24
Appliance method only	15	7	7	15	20	14
Rhythm only	19	14	14	20	20	32
Withdrawal only	11	7	12	7	11	20
All others and combinations	13	7	14	16	15	10

Even more pronounced trends are observed when pattern of use is investigated by marriage duration. The recently married are not only using contraception extensively, but are using effective methods. As many as 68 per cent are users, and 74 per cent of the recently married users were on oral pills, a level of use rarely seen in any group of women. If we allow for some discontinuation due to side effects or a decision to conceive, the extreme popularity of orals among newly married young females is highly evident. Another 13 per cent were on appliance methods and only four per cent relied on rhythm alone. This is surprising in view of the sizable number of Catholics that the group includes. Such extensive use of effective contraception if continued later in marriage should have a significant impact on fertility levels if only by reducing the number of unwanted pregnancies. At the very least it indicates widespread concern with spacing among the recently married.

Table 39 Percentage Currently Using Specified Types of Contraception by Marriage Duration

		Years Married					
	Total	*0–2*	*3–5*	*6–10*	*11–15*	*16–20*	*More than 20*
Number of Couples	1632	156	192	400	380	318	186
Number of Users	1022	107	113	271	243	204	84
Percentage of Non-Users	37	32	41	32	36	36	55
Percentage of Users	100	100	100	100	100	100	100
Oral pills only	47	74	58	47	43	33	43
Appliance methods only	25	13	15	25	26	34	33
Rhythm only	7	4	5	6	9	10	5
Withdrawal only	8	3	11	5	8	11	7
I.U.D. only	3	0	4	6	3	2	1
Combination of rhythm, withdrawal, and appliance	2	1	1	3	2	2	4
All others (douche, abstinence, chemical, etc.)	8	5	6	8	9	8	7

As in the case of age, use of orals decreases and use of appliance methods increases with marriage duration. However, as different cohorts of women are involved, the relationship cannot be generalized. The future contraceptive behaviour of the present young cohorts is unpredictable especially in view of developments in technology.

The only satisfactory way to resolve this question is by a longitudinal investigation which also is the only way generally to test explanatory hypotheses.

Education

As we have seen the use of contraception is positively associated with education (table 33). In a situation where organized programs purveying sophisticated birth control methods are reaching relatively few users, that is, where most users are on their own with respect to obtaining contraception, one might expect that education would be associated with the use of the most sophisticated methods, especially those requiring medical supervision. In addition to the general positive association between education and the adoption of innovative technology, there is the previously observed fact that the more educated women want fewer children than less educated women and thus would be attracted to a method, such as oral contraception, that offers a high degree of protection. These suppositions are borne out to a degree by the data in table 40. There are some irregularities which suggest that the relationship may be somewhat more complicated than our simple formulation or else that the irregularities, for example among Protestants, might be due to age or parity differences. It is certainly true that those with the least amount of education are the least likely to use orals. Over one-third, in fact, depend upon rhythm or withdrawal. We have previously noted that proportionately fewer of this group are users. So at the extremes, education is related both to extent and kind of use. At levels of education beyond the eighth grade, however, the use of oral contraception does not increase with education. There is an apparent trade-off among Protestants between the use of orals and appliance methods whereas among Catholics this is not the case, possibly because, as we shall see, the average length of oral use is less among Catholics. As the period since adoption lengthens, the opportunity for attrition also increases. As with most innovations and as is true of epidemiologic phenomena generally the curve of adoption for orals is characterized by rapid initial acceleration to a peak level of acceptance after which use may decline to a somewhat lower long-term prevalence rate. The alternative for women who discontinue the use of oral contraception is of course not nonuse but some other effective method. Of those who stopped use of orals for reasons other than to get pregnant almost 95 per cent switched to other methods of contraception. Two-thirds of these women shifted to effective methods such as the condom, diaphragm, and the I.U.D.

Figure 1 Percentage Distribution of Current Users by Specific Methods of Contraception and Wife's Religion

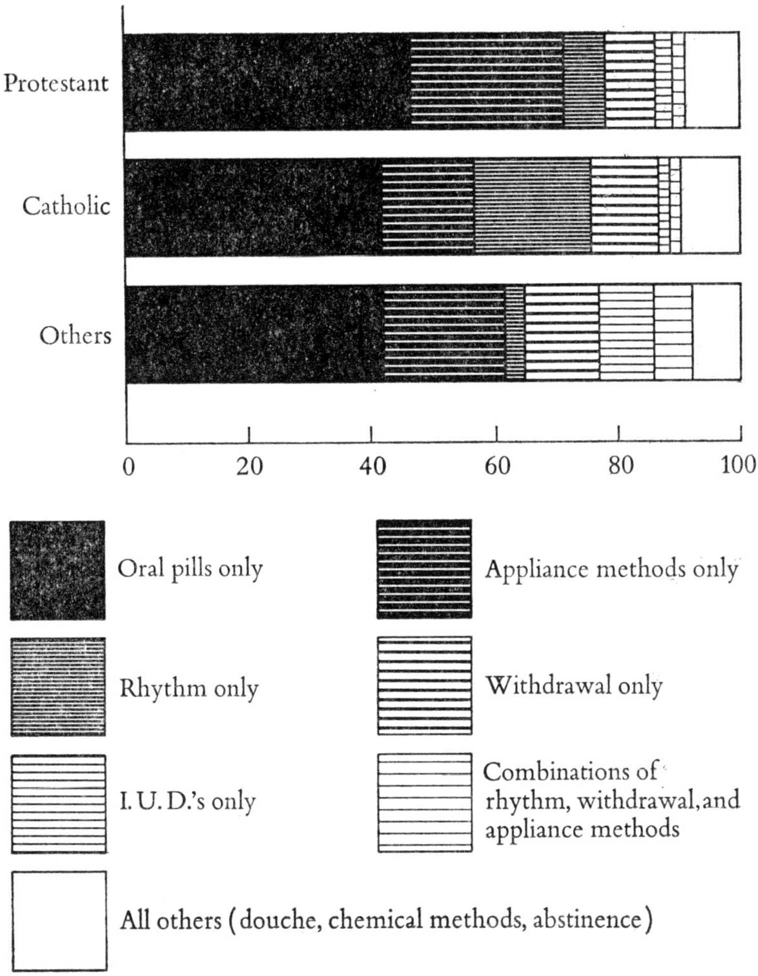

Table 40 Percentage of Users Adopting Specified Types of Contraception by Wife's Education and Religion

Type	*Total*	*8th Grade or less*	*9–11 years*	*12–13 years*	*College*
			TOTAL		
Number of Users	1022	156	411	316	130
Percentage of Users	100	100	100	100	100
Oral pills only	47	30	51	50	47
Appliance methods only	25	19	26	24	34
Rhythm only	7	14	6	6	6
Withdrawal only	8	24	6	4	1
All others and combinations	13	13	11	16	12
			PROTESTANTS		
Number of Users	677	57	295	232	93
Percentage of Users	100	100	100	100	100
Oral pills only	50	40	53	50	42
Appliance methods only	30	21	30	27	44
Rhythm only	3	9	2	5	1
Withdrawal only	5	16	6	5	0
All others and combinations	12	14	9	13	13
			CATHOLICS		
Number of Users	252	80	87	59	26
Percentage of Users	100	100	100	100	100
Oral pills only	42	23	47	54	54
Appliance methods only	15	20	13	14	8
Rhythm only	19	19	20	14	27
Withdrawal only	11	27	7	0	4
All others and combinations	13	11	13	18	7

Figure 2 Percentage Distribution of Current Users by Specific Methods of Contraception and Marriage Duration

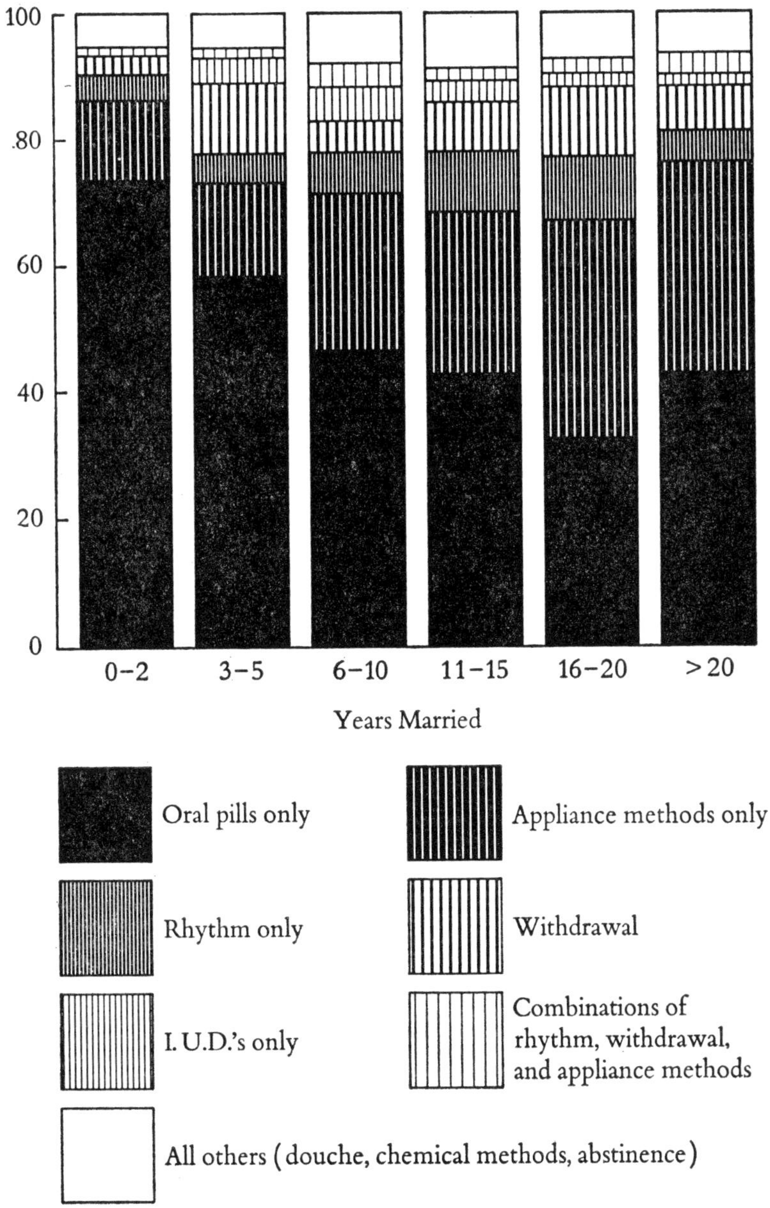

Unwanted Pregnancies[4]

Having looked at the extent of use and the types of contraceptive methods used, it remains to see how much success or failure couples have in achieving their fertility desires. Where actual performance falls below the desired level, given that the couple has been married a long enough time, the fault may be laid generally to sterility or subfecundity. But where actual performance exceeds the desired level, the main reason generally is contraceptive failure. In this section we will be concerned with the consequence of contraceptive failure, excess fertility. In order to eliminate the complicating factor of abortion and miscarriage, only those respondents whose pregnancies equal the actual number of children surviving at the time of the interview are considered in the present analysis. These respondents were asked: "Did your last pregnancy occur because you intentionally tried to have a child at that time?" Those who answered "no" to the above question were further asked, "At that time would you and your husband have preferred to have your pregnancy earlier, sometime later, or to have avoided it altogether?" Those who answered that they would have preferred to avoid the last child altogether are classified here as having had an unwanted child. Thus the concept refers to number failure and not spacing failure. It should be realized that this measure is based only on the last child, and does not include pregnancies some of which, especially for higher parity women, might also have been unwanted.

The percentage whose last child was unwanted is shown by parity and religion in table 41 as the percentage of the total in each group. The proportion reporting an unwanted child increases steadily with parity both among Catholics and non-Catholics. While for the first and second parity, the proportion reporting an unwanted birth is low and comparable for Catholics and non-Catholics, for higher parities, non-Catholics report substantially more unwanted pregnancies. This is because more of the high parity Catholics really desire larger families, whereas a good many non-Catholics attain these parities in spite of their desire to check the size of the family at a lower level.

[4] An extensive analysis of unwanted pregnancies in this sample was made by George Parakulam in his Master's thesis, "Wives Who Have Unwanted Children."

Summary

There is widespread approval of family planning. Even among the Catholics, 66 per cent approved of contraception and another 15 per cent gave it qualified approval.

Use of contraception is also high. 86 per cent of fecund women have used contraception at some time and more than two-thirds were using it at the time of the survey. Level of use does not vary very much by age or marriage duration, except that women 40 and over and those married 21 years or more appear to be below average both in current use and ever use. In part this is due to their higher prevalence of infecundity. The generally high level of use at all ages and marriage durations is indicative of widespread interest in spacing as well as in the limitation of births.

While contraceptive use does not vary much by age or duration, type of method does. Thus in a developed society where high levels of use are pervasive, motivational differences towards the use of contraception which are conditional by the couples' life cycle and family building situation, are expressed in the type of method used rather than in use or nonuse.

Table 41 Percentage of Wives Reporting Last Child as Unwanted by Parity and Religion of Wife

	CATHOLIC		NON-CATHOLIC	
Parity	*Percentage*	*Number*	*Percentage*	*Number*
1	6.90	87	6.13	212
2	5.96	151	6.70	358
3	12.96	108	21.97	223
4	27.27	66	41.00	100
5+	36.00	50	55.07	69
Mean/Total	14.07	462	17.15	962

Socio-economic characteristics show some relation to contraceptive use. Catholics, women in lower educational groups, the foreign born, and women whose husbands are blue collar workers are less likely to use contraception. Inclusion of foreign-born women in this list of below average users is puzzling since foreign-born women in this sample do not in general have high fertility.

Analysis of the methods used demonstrates the great popularity of oral contraception. Almost half of all users are on oral pills.

Chemical methods have become almost insignificant and non-mechanical methods such as rhythm and withdrawal are less often used among married couples. United States data would suggest that withdrawal might be widely used among young unmarried women. Use of orals is high even among Catholics with as many as 42 per cent of the Catholics who use any type of contraception using oral contraception exclusively. In the case of interfaith marriages, the wife's religious affiliation seems to be more important than the husband's in the choice of the contraceptive. Mixed Protestant–Catholic marriages are characterized by higher levels of use and by greater use of orals than marriages where both partners are Catholic. Again it is the wife's religion which seems to count most with respect to contraceptive behaviour.

Age and marriage duration are related to the type of contraceptive used. The popularity of the orals decreases with the age of the wife and consequently with marriage duration. Use of orals is also lower in the lower educational groups.

About one in five Catholic couples using contraception use the rhythm method. This figure becomes almost one in three among Catholic women 40 and over. There is evidence that prior to the advent of oral contraception these figures were substantially higher since many Catholic oral users formerly relied on rhythm.

Unwanted or excess fertility, excluding timing failures, is fairly substantial in view of the high levels of contraceptive use and in view of the social and psychological cost this often entails.

5

Oral Contraception[1]

We saw in the last chapter that oral contraception is the most popular method currently being used. Of the 1,632 married women in the sample, 752 women or 46 per cent have used oral pills sometime and 472 or 33 per cent were users at the time of the survey. In Canada, oral contraceptives first became available on a prescription basis in March 1961. The manufacturer currently enjoying the largest sales volume did not enter the market until February 1963. Yet, by the end of 1967, about half the married women exposed to the risk of pregnancy in a major metropolitan area were using oral contraception. This is a spectacular increase in the popularity of a medical innovation without benefit of large-scale programs or a panoply of market research and mass advertising and involving changes in long-established patterns of behaviour—all in a six year period.

Trends in Oral Contraceptive Use

The particular configuration of growth of oral usage is important for

[1] Parts of this chapter were published earlier in three articles. See Allingham, Balakrishnan, and Kantner, "Time Series of Growth in Use of Oral Contraceptives and the Differential Diffusion of Oral Anovulants"; Allingham, Balakrishnan, Kantner, "The End of Rapid Increase in the Use of Oral Anovulants? Some Problems in the Interpretation of Time Series of Oral Use Among Married Women"; Balakrishnan, Allingham, Kantner, "Analysis of Oral Contraceptive Use Through Multiple Decrement Life Table Techniques," *Demography*, 7, no. 4 (1970): 450-65.

the light it may throw on the possible impact of oral contraception on fertility during the 1960s and for what it may reveal about patterns of acceptance.

For a time-trend analysis of use it would have been advisable to have longitudinal samples. In the absence of longitudinal data we are forced to look retrospectively into the contraceptive use history of the cross sectional sample of women. Using such retrospective data the growth in popularity of oral contraception in the United States has been sketched by Ryder and Westoff.[2] For each month from January 1960 to September 1965, they calculated the proportion of women born since 1920 and married in or before the month concerned who were using oral anovulants. The resulting time series provides us with the first evidence of the growth configuration of oral contraception in a developed country. Their data show a consistent increase.

Aggregate growth curves for the Toronto sample and for the U.S. are shown in figure 3. The first time series for Toronto women, presented in the light solid line, is constructed in a manner identical to the Ryder–Westoff series for the U.S. which is shown as a broken line.[3] The level of each month of the year represents the proportion of once-married women with husbands present, using the pill in that month. The denominator increases each month as women married in that month join the population. Thus, the denominator approximates a population at risk in that non-married women are excluded and the remaining women are aged 45 and under. However, a proportion of these women in any month will not be a risk because of pregnancy or sterility. The denominator is thus inflated. The growth curve in figure 3 illustrated by the dotted line is constructed by excluding from the population at risk women who were sub-fecund.[4] Ideally,

[2] Ryder and Westoff, *Reproduction in the United States, 1965*, Chapter 6 and Westoff, ed., *Toward the End of Growth*, Chapter 3.

[3] The women were presented a monthly calendar going back to 1959 and were asked to note the months in each year that they used the pill (see Appendix A for questionnaire). As the series are constructed retrospectively certain biases due to changing age and marriage durations are introduced which are discussed later in the chapter. This will naturally affect some of the comparisons with the U.S. data which are also constructed retrospectively. However, these biases are unlikely to be large enough to affect basic patterns of use.

[4] The women retained in the population at risk were those who replied "No" to the question: "Is there any reason why you and your husband could not have another child if you wanted to?" Our population at risk is, therefore, comprised of women who were not, to their knowledge, sub-fecund (or whose marriages were not, to their knowledge, sub-fecund) at the time of the interview. However, our control is imperfect in that some previous

women pregnant at any point in the series would also be excluded for the period of their pregnancy and for some time thereafter, to cover the period of post-partum amenorrhea, but such a refinement is not undertaken here. The population "at risk" in the remainder of this analysis of the growth trend consists of once-married women, living with their husbands, under 46 years of age, whose marriages are not, to their knowledge, sub-fecund.

Education, Religion, and the Adoption of Oral Contraception

Because of the attitudes of the Roman Catholic Church on oral contraception, other things being equal, a lower rate of oral usage would be expected among Catholic women at risk than among Protestant women. We have seen in the last chapter that this is true with respect to current use. Yet we also have seen that more Catholics use orals than any other method and that the proportion using orals approaches the levels of use among non-Catholics. But what about the pattern of adoption? The moral status of the pill was not clearly defined during this period and oral use, therefore, could perhaps be more easily rationalized.[5] There was in fact some currency given to the doctrine of "probabilism" which before "Humanae Vitae" squelched the notion, held that approval of oral contraception by the Church was probable given the great pressure on the Vatican towards that end and the theological argument which had been marshalled on behalf of the pill. Therefore, for a Catholic in doubt about what method to use, adoption of orals would probably turn out to be morally sanctioned. This as we now know, turned out to be a philosophical will-o'-the-wisp. Nevertheless, there were ideas in the air which gave support to Catholic couples eager to take up this new method. There was at the same time reason to hesitate and to wait for papal clarification. The resolution of this moral quandary could be expected to differ by education since the better educated Catholics have been shown to be more concerned with matters of doctrine. Moreover, innovations are more likely to become known, and if

sub-fecundity, cured by the time of the survey, might have existed and not all sub-fecund women at the time of the survey would have been sub-fecund over the entire span of our series. In addition, women pregnant at any point in the series have not been excluded.

[5] The papal encyclical Humanae Vitae, dated 25 July 1968 and subsequent to our survey, made rationalization of pill use more difficult. A higher proportion of Roman Catholic than Protestant women reported use of the pill for "medical reasons" in the latest American survey, as well as in our own. See Ryder and Westoff, "Use of Oral Contraception in the United States, 1965."

Figure 3 Oral Use among Once Married Women, under Age 46 at End of Series and Living with Husband—Toronto and the United States *

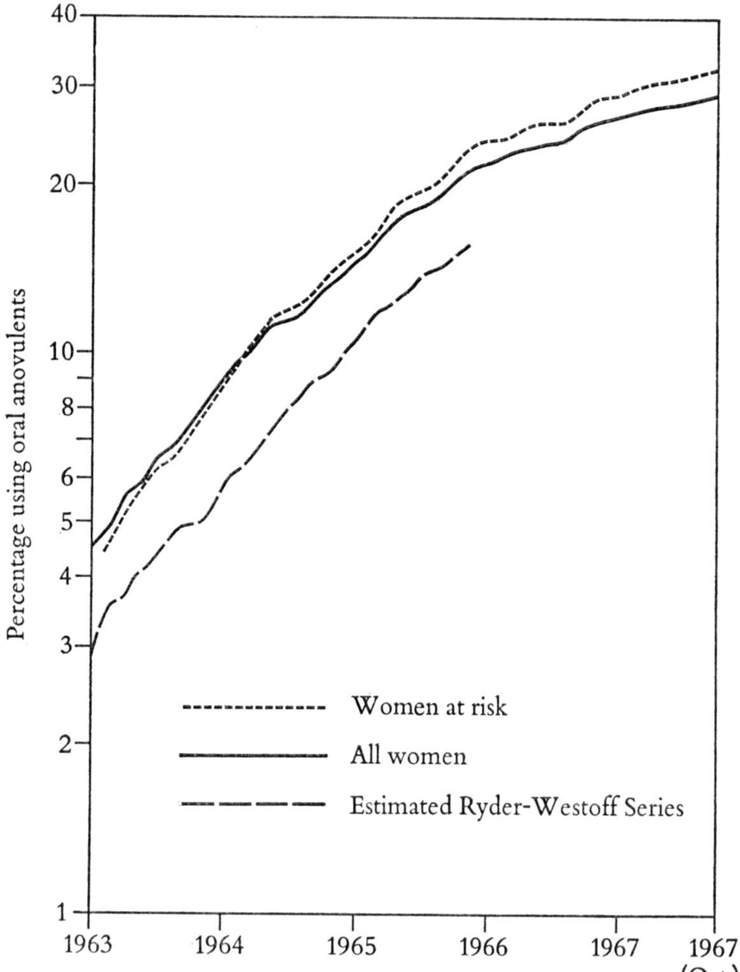

* All series shown are semi-logarithmic. Percentages to plot the Ryder-Westoff series were estimated from the non-logarithmic growth curve in Ryder and Westoff, op. cit., Figure 1, p. 2. The lower use level of the Ryder-Westoff series is what one would expect between a national sample and an urban sample.

thought desirable, to be adopted by the better educated. Other things being equal, then, we might expect oral contraception to have been adopted first by more educated women.

Figure 4 and table 42 present growth rates of oral contraceptive usage for women by religion and two broad educational categories: less than grade 12, and grade 12 or more.

Among Protestant women, education appears to be of negligible importance for either the level of use or the growth rate of use. From mid-1965 to the beginning of 1967, the level of use or the rate at which use increased among better educated Protestant women is slightly higher, but convergence is apparent as one moves into 1967. A levelling off in the rate of growth for both categories of Protestant women is also evident from the beginning of 1966, approaching an apparent plateau in 1967.

While the numbers of Roman Catholic women in either educational category are too small in the early months of the series to allow any confident conclusions, the pattern does suggest a somewhat later start with orals among better educated Catholics, but a much faster rate of growth. Such a pattern would be consistent with the notion that better educated Catholics went through an initial period of doubt and hesitation followed by rapid adoption beginning in late 1965 as the doctrine of probabilism became more credible. The level of use among more highly educated Catholics approaches that of less educated Catholics in the latter part of 1965 and continues upward at an impressive rate from that point on ultimately equalling the level of use among Protestants. The rate of growth for less educated Catholic women levels off substantially from the rate sustained until 1965. The rapid rate of increase in oral use among Catholics, observed throughout 1964 and 1965 begins to falter in 1966, levelling off considerably during 1967. A similar levelling process may be observed in figure 4 for Protestants. That little of this levelling off in the growth rate of oral use can be attributed to the changing marriage duration distribution over the series is shown later in this chapter.

A comparison of the series on figure 4 reveals important differences in the diffusion of oral contraception among Protestant and Roman Catholic women. By late 1963, over ten per cent of Protestant women in both educational categories were using the pill. The corresponding level of use among Roman Catholic women is not attained until the early part of 1965. Yet, by the time ten per cent of Catholic women were using orals, over 20 per cent of Protestant women were on the pill.

Figure 4 Oral Use among Once Married Fecund Women * by Religion and Education

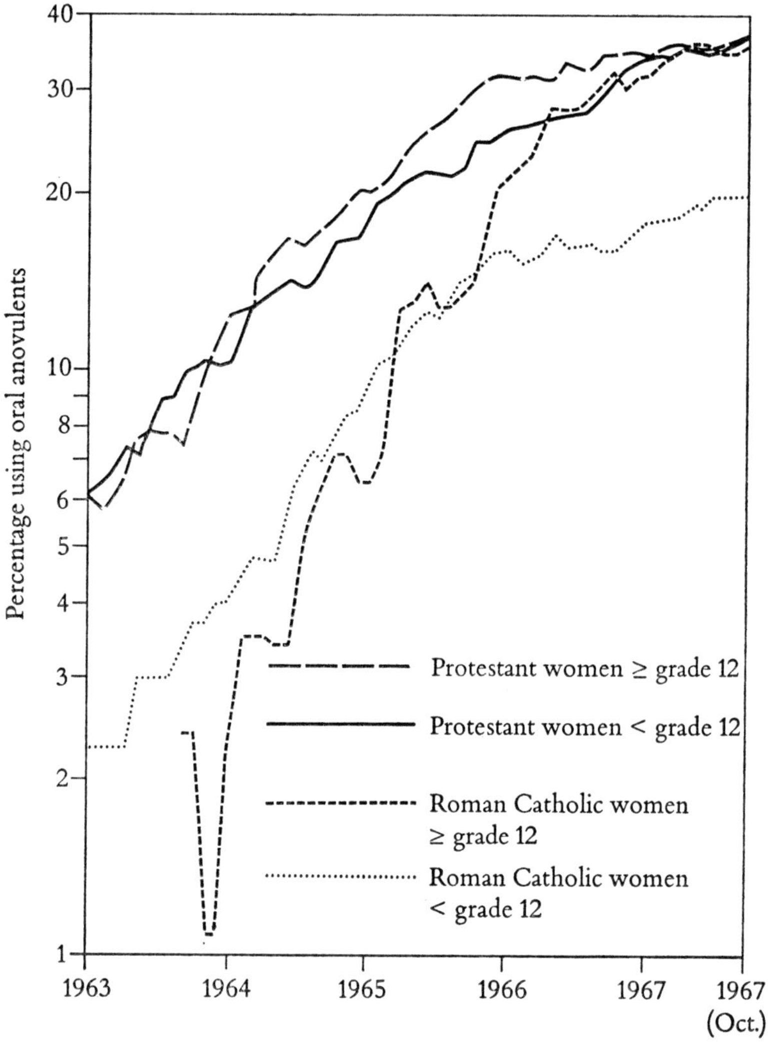

* Aged under 46 at end of series, living with husband and no reported subfecundity at time of interview.

The early lag in use by Roman Catholic women of both educational categories and the early "peaking" of use among the less educated Catholics, combine to leave Catholic women in the aggregate below Protestant women in level of use at the end of the series. However, because of a tremendous rate of increase in use throughout 1966, the more highly educated Roman Catholics catch up to both Protestant groups by early 1967. Therefore, by the latter part of 1967, more highly educated Catholic women were as likely as either category of Protestant women to be using oral anovulants.

National Origin

About 60 per cent of the Roman Catholic women at the terminal point of the series are foreign born. However, just over half the Catholic women with grade 12 or more education are foreign born compared to 63 per cent of the less educated. In particular, there is a heavy Italian-born component among the less-educated Roman Catholics.[6] There is therefore a possibility that national origin is responsible for some of the difference shown in figure 4 between educated and less well-educated Catholics. Figure 5 supports this suggestion. Use of oral contraception among foreign-born Catholics with less than 12 years of education is very much lower than it is for native-born Catholics with the same education. At the end of the series in figure 5, only about ten per cent of foreign-born Catholics with less than grade 12 education are on the pill in contrast to over 35 per cent of the native born in the same educational category—about the same percentage as found among the more highly educated Roman Catholics in figure 4. The striking difference between native and foreign-born women with less than 12 years of education is in the level of use rather than the pattern of adoption, for the slopes of the diffusion curves are fairly similar.

The series by national origin for Roman Catholic women of grade 12 or more education goes back only to July 1965 because of the very small sample size before that date. Figure 5 suggests that national origin discriminates for oral use less among better educated Catholic women than among the less educated. Our sample is too small to pursue the ethnicity issue further.

Figure 6 suggests that although national origin discriminates among Protestant women, it is not an important factor in the com-

[6] One-third of our Roman Catholic women with less than grade 12 education are Italian born in contrast to about four percent of those with grade 12 or more education.

Table 42 Use of Oral Contraception by Month and Year among Once Married Fecund Women *
by Religion and Education

Month† and Year of Use	ALL AT RISK		PROTESTANT				ROMAN CATHOLIC			
			Less than Grade 12		*Grade 12 and above*		*Less than Grade 12*		*Grade 12 and above*	
	Percentage Using Orals	*Base Population*	*Percentage Using Orals*	*Base Population*	*Percentage Using Orals*	*Base Population*	*Percentage Using Orals*	*Base Population*	*Percentage Using Orals*	*Base Population*
1963										
January	4.4	1,112	6.2	372	6.0	300	2.3	263	0.0	78
April	5.3	1,126	7.2	376	6.6	304	2.3	266	0.0	79
July	6.3	1,146	8.8	384	7.7	312	3.0	268	0.0	81
October	7.2	1,168	10.0	391	8.5	319	3.7	271	2.4	84
1964										
January	8.7	1,174	10.4	393	12.2	321	4.0	273	2.4	84
April	10.6	1,180	13.2	394	15.2	323	4.7	274	3.5	86
July	11.9	1,198	13.8	398	16.2	327	6.6	275	4.5	89
October	13.8	1,219	16.5	401	17.9	336	7.6	277	7.4	94
1965										
January	15.4	1,229	18.7	402	19.8	338	9.3	281	6.4	94
April	18.3	1,237	21.0	404	23.5	340	11.3	283	12.8	94
July	19.1	1,263	21.8	409	26.6	346	12.2	288	12.9	101
October	22.3	1,282	24.3	412	30.3	353	14.8	292	14.3	105

1966										
January	24.0	1,289	26.0	415	32.0	353	16.3	294	21.7	106
April	25.3	1,302	27.0	419	31.5	356	15.9	297	26.4	106
July	25.9	1,323	27.3	425	33.1	366	16.4	301	28.0	107
October	28.3	1,348	31.1	431	34.9	375	16.1	305	33.0	112
1967										
January	29.2	1,354	34.0	433	34.0	377	18.0	306	32.1	112
April	30.9	1,362	35.5	434	36.1	382	18.6	307	36.3	113
July	31.4	1,384	36.1	440	35.5	392	20.1	310	35.3	116
October	32.8	1,407	37.8	447	37.4	401	19.9	311	37.5	120

**Under 46 years of age at end of series, living with husband and no reported subfecundity at time of interview.*

†Refer to a particular month and not to be confused with a quarter.

The summation of base populations by religion and education above does not equal the "all at risk" column since Jews and other religions were included in the "all at risk" category.

Figure 5 Oral Use among Once Married Fecund Roman Catholic Women * by Nativity and Education

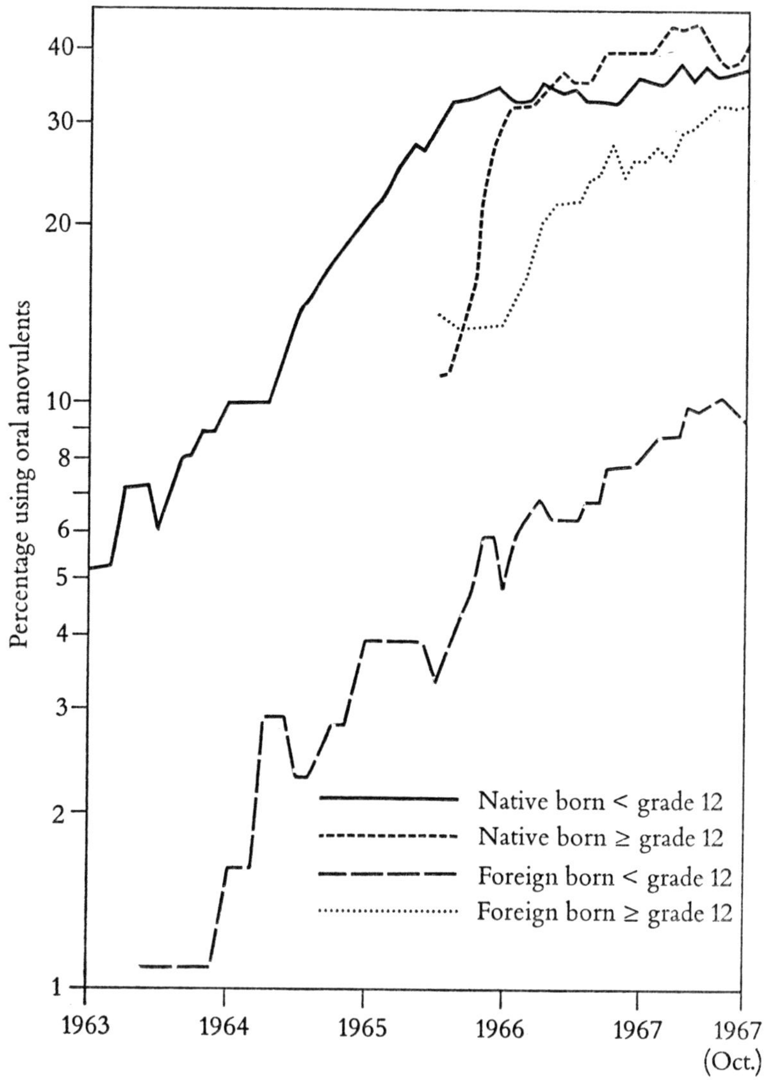

* Aged under 46 at end of series, living with husband and no reported subfecundity at time of interview.

position of aggregate time series for Protestant women shown in figure 4.

In terms of possible "biases" in the aggregate series shown in figure 3, the series in figure 4 suggests that shifts in the proportion of Roman Catholic women and in their educational distribution might influence an aggregate series. However, figure 5 shows that the series for Catholic women with less than grade 12 education takes its shape primarily through the heavy weighting of the foreign born. Any shift in the distribution of Roman Catholic women by education and national origin will, therefore, influence the aggregate series for Catholic women. Thus in addition to the bias introduced into aggregate time series due to changing composition by marriage duration, bias can also result from shifts in other compositional aspects such as nativity and education. This is especially true when dealing with data for a local population subject to significant migratory movements.

Bias Due to Marriage Duration

As noted, interpretation of time series on oral use is complicated by a changing marriage duration distribution over the series. As our sample is composed of women who were once married and under 46 years of age at the time of the survey, any assembly of data from the sample with respect to age and marital status for a time prior to the survey date changes the composition of the sample by truncation of the age distribution at its upper end and by the elimination of some women whose eligibility for the sample was established, that is, those who first married after the earlier date. A joint analysis by marriage duration and time period, using retrospective data such as undertaken here, must contend with this problem. It becomes more severe the farther back in time the analysis is pushed. Fortunately in this regard, our oral series covers only about a six year period—from the introduction of orals in Canada in 1961 to the end of 1967. Furthermore, we present here a foreshortened series, going back only to January 1963, which roughly dates the beginning of oral contraception as a widely known and available method.

The age bias which results when the oldest ages are truncated will be most evident in the highest marital duration categories. For this reason, except when marriage cohorts are being followed, the present analysis concentrates on the low duration groups which are relatively unaffected by age truncation. The bias due to changing marital status composition, on the other hand, has its main effect on low

Figure 6 Oral Use among Once Married Fecund Protestant Women * by Nativity and Education

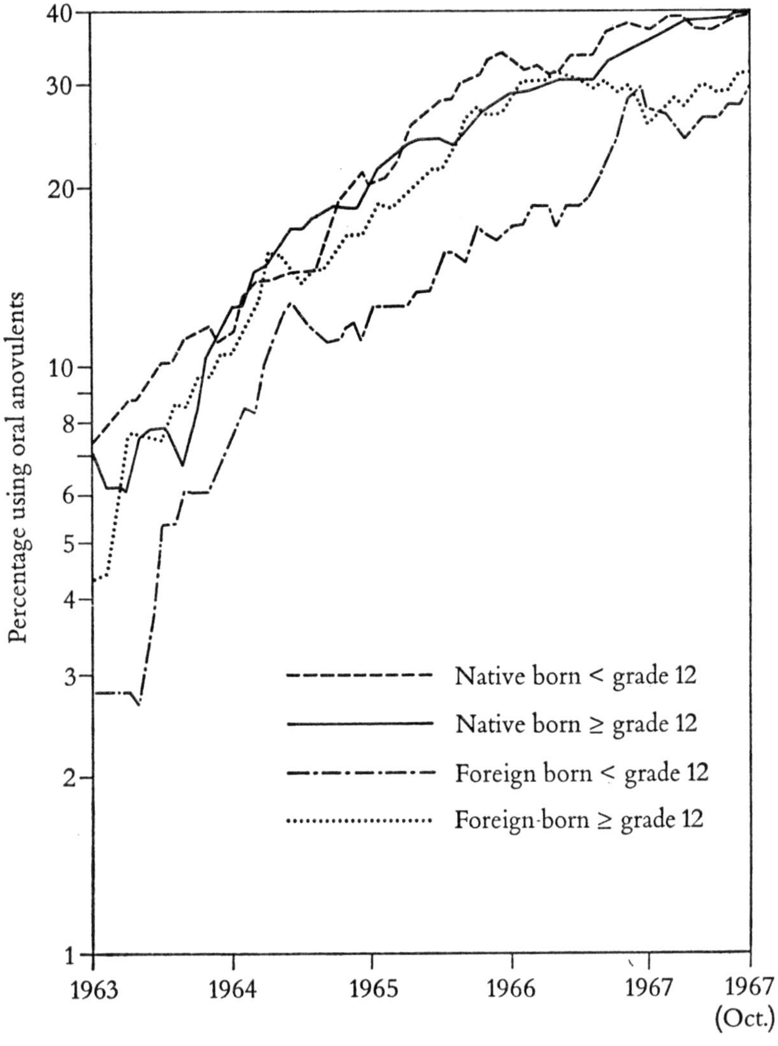

* Aged under 46 at end of series, living with husband and no reported subfecundity at time of interview.

duration groups. For example, the women from our sample who in 1966 were married less than twelve months differ from a sample of such women taken in 1961 to the extent that the latter group was added to or subtracted from, due to death, migration, or change of marital status, e.g., divorce. Mortality at these ages is too low to be an important source of bias. The degree to which bias results from migration or change in marital status will depend in part on the frequency of each type of event. The degree to which any such bias affects the analysis depends further on the extent to which these events are selective with respect to factors related to the use of oral contraception. While there is no basis for estimating the net result of these sources of bias, there is some likelihood that the effects may be offsetting. For example, migration streams flow in both directions and to some extent contain similar types of individuals. There are reasons also to suspect that the net effect due to changed marital status, essentially through divorce, is not great. While some couples who eventually become divorced may have an interest in a highly effective contraceptive such as the oral pill for the very reason that their marriage is tentative, others in the same situation may not feel the need for any form of contraception. The magnitude of shifts in marriage duration over the time series of use due to factors discussed above is provided in table 43.

One can deal with the problem of changing marital duration distributions in a series by standardizing on one distribution. However, any

Table 43 Marriage Duration Distributions of Women Married on or before Specified Dates

Marriage Duration Months	JANUARY *1963*	*1964*	*1965*	*1966*	*1967*	NOVEMBER *1967*
Total: Number	1323	1388	1446	1508	1574	1632
Percentage	100.0	100.0	100.0	100.0	100.0	100.0
Under 12	5.0	4.7	4.0	4.1	4.2	3.5
12–35	13.8	11.1	9.1	8.2	7.6	7.8
36–71	17.0	16.0	16.3	16.4	13.9	11.6
72–107	18.3	18.1	18.2	15.0	14.1	14.5
108–143	14.4	15.8	15.3	16.0	15.9	16.1
144–179	15.2	14.0	13.3	12.6	13.9	13.6
180–227	11.9	14.9	15.8	16.4	16.6	15.6
228 or more	4.4	5.4	8.0	11.3	13.8	17.3

decision on a standard distribution will have implications for the pattern of growth in oral usage observed over the series. For example, standardization on the 1963 marital duration distribution of table 43 will weight the duration-specific rates of the short duration categories more heavily than would standardization on the November 1967 distribution, possibly providing a quite different picture of oral usage.

The problem of bias and the need for standardization having been stated we now look at the trends in use with these considerations in mind. There is particular interest in the growth rate of oral usage in developed countries in the latter part of the 1960s since the tremendous rates of growth in the use of orals initially observed could not be maintained indefinitely. Will the level of oral use stabilize, and if so, at what level? Our data suggest that the period of rapid growth in oral usage had come to an end in 1966. However, from the above discussion of the possible impact or overall growth rates of the shifting marital duration distribution, it is evident that some of the falling off of the growth rate might be an artifact of a shifting marital duration distribution, in view of the popularity of oral contraception among young, recently married women.

Figure 7 illustrates the effect of standardizing the series on the 1963 and November 1967 distributions in table 43.

Standardizing on the 1963 marital duration distribution results in a less noticeable fall in the growth rate towards the end of the series. The reason is the combination of the greater weight of shorter duration categories with the faster rate of growth in oral use among the shorter duration women. Standardizing on the November 1967 distribution produces little change from the unstandardized series, since the aging of the unstandardized "cohort" produces a marital duration distribution resembling the November 1967 distribution. Moreover, the use rates over the early portion of the series do not vary greatly by duration. Since only the November 1967 distribution can be taken as representative of its population, standardization on that distribution is intuitively more appealing.

To determine whether there has been a change in the growth rate of oral usage among married women, one should look separately at growth rates of duration-specific categories and ideally consider trends in oral use within marriage cohorts. Figure 8 based on data for eight duration categories provides an illustration of somewhat different duration-specific trends. Approximate variance estimates for the rates reported can be calculated by applying the formula $s = \sqrt{p(1-p)/N}$, and using the base populations given in appendix D.

Only the shortest duration category in figure 8—that of 12 months

Figure 7 Oral Use among Once Married Women Showing Effect of Standardization for Marriage Duration (Semi-Logarithmic Scale)

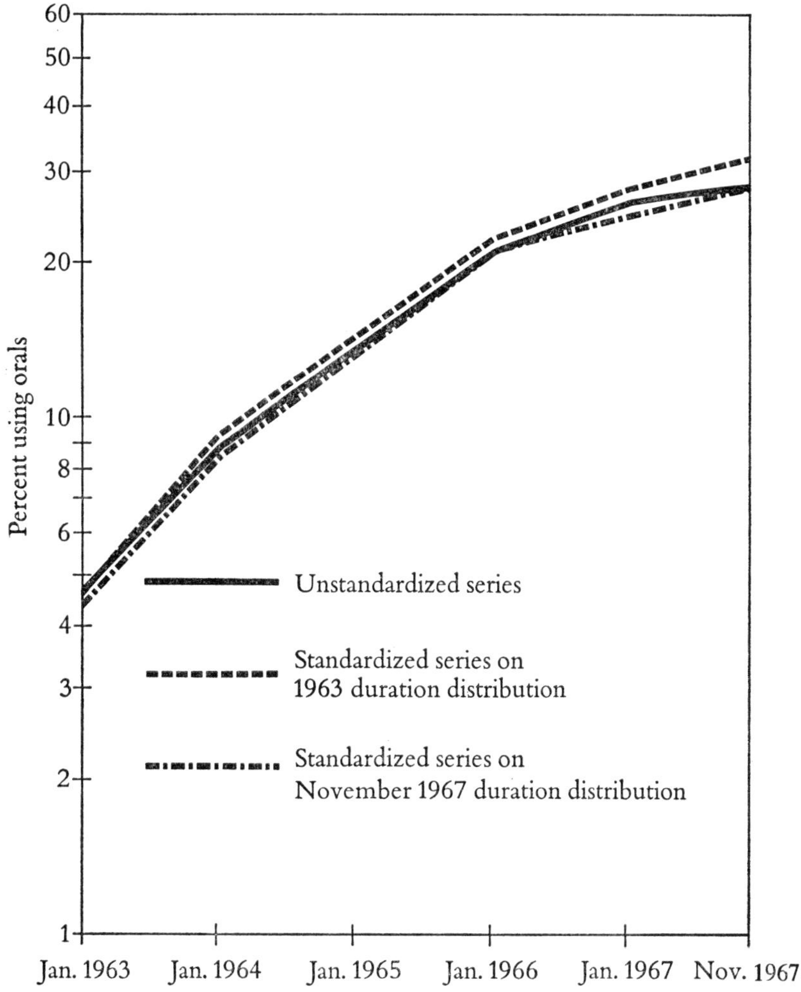

Figure 8 Use of Oral Contraception by Marital Duration

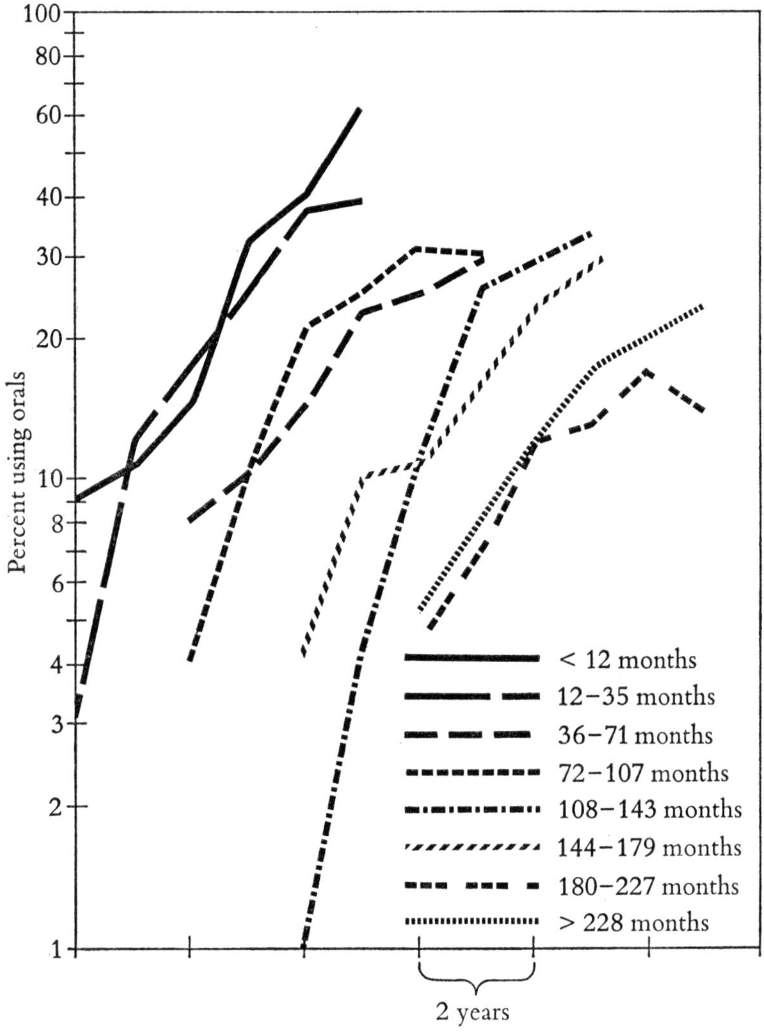

The horizontal axis is segmented into two year intervals. Duration specific series each cover a period of $4\frac{10}{12}$ years—from January 1963 to November 1967. For readability and convenience in plotting, series are paired and plotted so that the starting points (January 1963) shift to the right by 2 year intervals from lower to higher duration series.

or less shows an increased rate of oral use over the last segment of the series—January 1967 to November 1967. A marked decrease in the rate of increase during the last segment of the series is evident for four of the duration categories, with the break in growth rates for the remaining three categories first appearing in the second to last segment—after January 1966.

The duration-specific series of figure 8 suffers the weakness of being comprised at each observation point by women belonging to different marriage cohorts. The problem is analogous to that of a fertility series based on age-specific fertility rates derived from a single period. For example, the women comprising the duration category of 12 months or less in January 1963 are most likely different in many important respects from women comprising that duration category in November 1967. Ideally then, in order to evaluate trends in oral usage one should examine oral usage over time within separate marriage cohorts.

The oral use rates of the eight most recent marriage cohorts are plotted in figure 9. For the earliest marriage cohorts a crude projection provided estimates of use rates for durations of less than one year. (The rate of use at the last observation point was halved for each projected observation point. The results appear reasonable in view of the introduction of orals in 1961.)

Although the data for some of the eight cohorts cover a very limited period, the series do not suggest an increase in the growth rate of oral usage among married women even though the overall percentage of married women using orals is expected to increase towards the use level of the latest marriage cohort.

Returning to figure 7 which shows the growth curve for usage among all women regardless of marriage duration or cohort, it is apparent that the curve is convex for two reasons: first, the ever higher use rates of the new marriage cohorts, and second, the rapid adoption of orals among earlier marriage cohorts at later duration. This latter factor has become less important as use levels appear to stabilize around 30 per cent. While any attempt to project future levels of oral usage would be presumptuous, the above trends together with the analysis of plans for future use presented later in this chapter suggest that we have most likely seen the end of rapid increase in the use of oral anovulants for the population under consideration.

Past Contraceptive Practices of Current Oral Users

A crucial question in connection with the impact of the "pill" on fer-

Figure 9 Use of Oral Contraception by Marriage Cohort

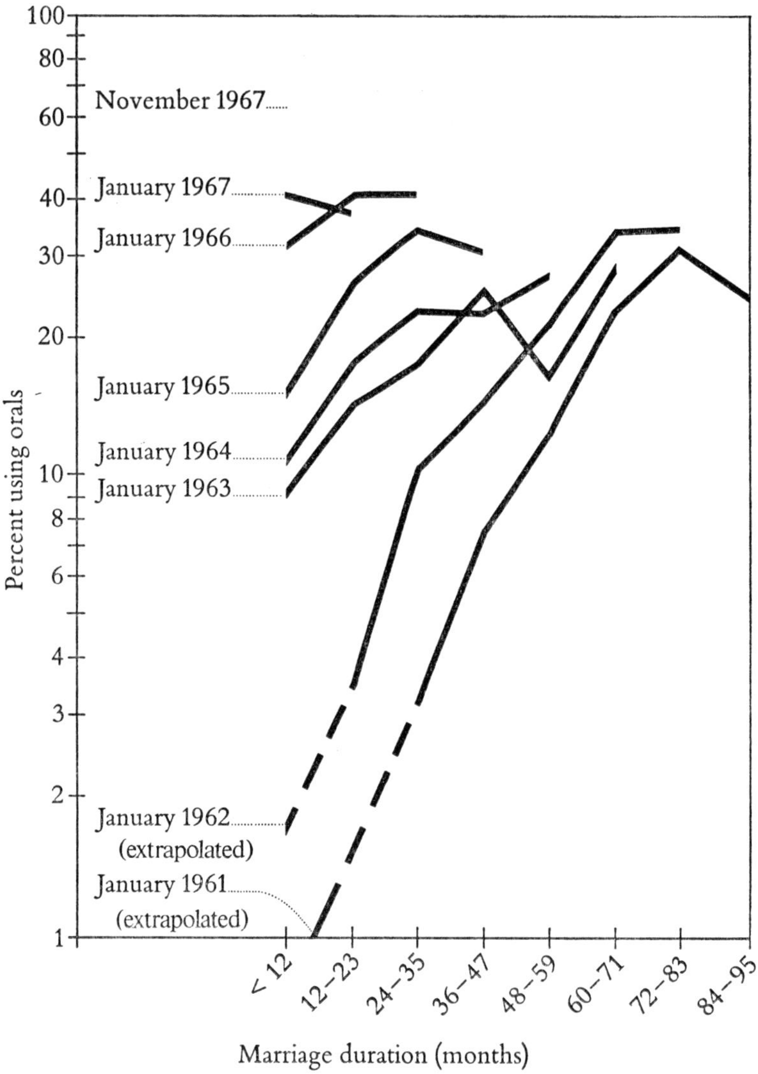

tility since 1960 concerns the methods of contraception in use prior to its adoption.[7] Popular thinking on the subject and even some unguarded professional speculation has assumed that the introduction of orals has substantially reduced the risk of unwanted pregnancy. This may well be so, but to our knowledge the point has not been demonstrated. Indeed, the opposite has been suggested by Westoff and Ryder who from an overall comparison of pre and post pill distributions showing the use of conventional methods conclude that "the pill is more likely than not to be a replacement for the condom or the diaphragm, both highly effective contraceptives."[8] However, data showing declines in the proportion of condom and diaphragm users from 1960 to 1965 along with growing use of orals, while highly suggestive, are less satisfactory than a case-by-case examination of the methods used by married women prior to their adoption of oral contraception. Such an examination is the focus of the remainder of this section.

Most of the women (77 per cent) now using the pill had used another method previously (table 44). For this sizeable group therefore, adoption of oral contraception reduced the risk of unwanted pregnancy to the extent that the pill is more efficient than the methods it supplanted. The remaining 23 per cent of our sample of oral users are women for whom the pill was their first method. Since the bulk of this group was married in 1960 or later, they were able to elect the pill over other methods which they otherwise might have used. Adoption of orals by this group reduced their risk of unwanted pregnancy to the extent that the pill is more efficient than the method that might have been used in its absence.[9]

[7] For women whose first method was the pill, it would be necessary in assessing the impact of oral contraception to impute a pre-pill level of risk. Other aspects of the problem have to do with the growth in use of the pill since its introduction and the continuation rates associated with it.

[8] Ryder and Westoff, "The United States: The Pill and the Birth Rate, 1960–1965," p. 3. However, their analysis of change from 1965 to 1970 shows a marked reduction in unwanted pregnancy the credit for which they give to the "contraceptive revolution" led by a continued rise in the popularity of orals which increased from 24 per cent in 1965 to 34 per cent in 1970. See Ryder and Westoff, "Wanted and Unwanted Fertility in the United States: 1965 and 1970."

[9] Some additional allowance needs to be made for the possibility that orals are somewhat more acceptable to recently married women and thus might increase their overall use of contraception. Problems of this sort suggest the utility of cohort analysis in dealing with the adoption of innovations which are related to the life cycle. This point was made to the authors originally by Professor Dudley Kirk.

Table 44 Current Oral Contraceptors According to Previous Use Status, Parity, and Religion*

Religion and Parity	*Used a Method Previously*	*No Method Previously*	*Total Per Cent*	*N*†
All Religions				
All parities	77	23	100	463
0	33	67	100	60
1–2	75	25	100	210
3	89	11	100	90
4+	95	5	100	103
Protestant				
All parities	76	24	100	321
0	30	70	100	43
1–2	76	24	100	138
3+	92	8	100	140
Roman Catholic				
All parities	76	24	100	104
0	—	—	100	11
1–2	65	35	100	49
3+	98	2	100	42

**Excludes use "for medical purposes."*
†*Sub-totals may not add to grand total because of item Non-Response.*

The major variation in previous use status, shown in tables 44 and 45, is related to presumed stages in the family cycle. Thus, low parity women and those recently married are less likely to have used another method previously. Interestingly there is little variation in previous use status by religion, partly it may be supposed, because we are dealing here with women who are current users. As we shall see in the following section, however, there are significant differences in the switching patterns behind these gross similarities. The differences in previous use by education (table 46) are no doubt produced in large measure by differences in age and parity. Less educated women in the sample tend to be slightly older and thus would have greater opportunity to have used a previous method—and more reason since they are of somewhat high average parity. Again, Protestant–Catholic differences are slight.

A detailed analysis of switching patterns is afforded by the data in table 47 which shows the method last used by women currently using orals. The condom and diaphragm, in that order, account for over half (59 per cent) of previous methods. If we add to this figure the proportion using various spermicides and the I.U.D., 70 per cent of women who had previously used a method had been using relatively efficient methods in contrast to 27 per cent who switched to orals from the relatively inefficient methods of rhythm or withdrawal.

There are differences according to parity in the method last used. The most reliable and systematic of these is the apparent shift from condom to diaphragm as parity increases. By education the switching patterns do not vary significantly beyond the elementary level. Women whose education does not go beyond the eighth grade showed a somewhat greater preference for withdrawal and simple intravaginal methods before adopting the pill. Since differences by education may reflect differences in age and other relevant variables, it is hazardous to push the analysis further at this point.

Table 45 Current Oral Contraceptors According to Previous Use Status, Marriage Date, and Religion*

Religion and Marriage Date	*Used a Method Previously*	*No Method Previously*	*Total Per Cent*	*N*†
All Religions				
1949 or before	95	5	100	62
1950–54	95	5	100	75
1955–59	93	7	100	124
1960–64	72	28	100	110
1965 and later	33	67	100	88
Protestant				
1954 or before	94	6	100	107
1955–59	91	9	100	86
1960 and later	53	47	100	127
Roman Catholic				
1954 or before	100	0	100	23
1955–59	100	0	100	27
1960 and later	54	46	100	52

**Excludes use "for medical purposes."*
†*Sub-totals do not add to grand total because of item Non-Response.*

Not unexpectedly, the patterns of previous use are associated with religious differences (table 48) and in a manner that has implications for the relative impact of the change to orals. Whereas only 18 per cent of Protestants switched to the pill from rhythm and withdrawal,

56 per cent of our Roman Catholic sample made the change. While it would be expected that a large proportion of Catholics who switched to orals would do so from the rhythm method, the shift was actually disproportionate. Whereas 23 per cent of Catholic women using contraception were either using the rhythm method currently or had used it prior to orals, former rhythm users contributed 44 per cent of the current oral users. It would seem that among current users of oral contraceptives, the effect of switching has been to reduce the risk of unwanted pregnancy considerably more for Roman Catholics than for Protestants.

Table 46 Current Oral Contraceptors According to Previous Use Status, Education, and Religion*

Religion and Education	*Used a Method Previously*	*No Method Previously*	*Total Per Cent*	*N*†
All Religions				
Grade 8 or less	84	16	100	44
Grade 9–11	78	22	100	198
Grade 12	79	21	100	108
Grade 13+	72	28	100	79
University degree	62	38	100	29
Protestant				
Grade 8 or less	85	15	100	20
Grade 9–11	79	21	100	150
Grade 12	77	23	100	79
Grade 13+ University degree	70	30	100	70
Roman Catholic				
Grade 8 or less	90	10	100	20
Grade 9–11	78	22	100	37
Grade 12	78	22	100	23
Grade 13+ University degree	59	41	100	22

**Excludes use "for medical purposes."*
†*Sub-totals may not all add to grand total because of item Non-Response.*

The reduction in risk of pregnancy among pill using Roman Catholics is considerable for all parities. High parity (3+) Roman Catholics enjoyed the greatest decline in risk with nearly two-thirds changing from rhythm or withdrawal. Among Protestants there is little

Table 47 Method Previously Used by Current Oral Contraceptors*

	Rhythm	With-drawal	Dia-phragm	Vaginal Prepara-tions	Condom	I.U.D.	Other Methods	Total Per Cent	N†
All Current Users	17.1	10.0	25.9	9.1	33.3	1.4	3.1	100.0	351
Parity 1–2	18.5	10.2	19.1	8.9	39.5	0.6	3.2	100.0	157
Parity 3	7.7	15.4	35.9	10.3	23.1	2.6	5.1	100.0	78
Parity 4+	24.5	5.1	32.7	9.2	24.5	2.0	2.0	100.0	98
Education									
Grade 8 and below	13.5	18.9	16.2	13.5	29.7	5.4	2.7	100.0	37
Grade 9–11	17.4	9.0	25.8	8.4	34.2	0.6	4.5	100.0	155
Grade 12	17.9	8.3	28.6	7.1	33.3	2.4	2.4	100.0	81
Grade 13 or more	15.8	9.2	27.6	10.5	32.9	0.0	3.9	100.0	76

**Excludes use "for medical purposes."*
†Sub-totals do not add to grand total because of item Non-Response.
Zero parity not shown.

difference in the distribution by parity group that does not appear to be explainable as a function of the condom to diaphragm shift.

In order to assess the probable impact of oral contraception on fertility in the sixties one must not only examine the previous use status of current oral users, but also the duration of pill use (table 49). Of current users of oral contraceptives in our sample who had used another method, about 35 per cent had switched to orals prior to January 1965.[10] A slightly larger proportion of Protestants (38 per cent) than Catholics (27 per cent) switched prior to that date. This delay in adoption by Roman Catholics would tend to offset partially the gains in protection implied by their switching from relatively inefficient methods. The impact of oral contraception on Roman Catholics is therefore more recent than for Protestants but more efficient in terms of method substitution.

Roman Catholics who did switch to the pill prior to January 1965 were somewhat more likely than those who changed later to switch from relatively efficient methods, a fact which is consistent with the notion of the "probabilistic" argument. The previous use profile of Protestants is generally similar regardless of when the switch was made except with respect to use of the condom and diaphragm—a difference which suggests a parity effect.

The small number of Roman Catholics in each marriage duration category (table 50) precludes much comment on those distributions. The high proportion switching from the condom among Roman Catholics married in 1960 or later suggests that we may be picking up a favourite pre-marital method. The same might be true for Protestants although the condom appears to retain its popularity to a greater degree among Protestants. Otherwise, Protestants exhibit a decrease in the proportion using withdrawal and an increase in the proportion using the diaphragm as marriage duration increases. This may reflect a move to more efficient methods with increasing parity. Apart from these differences the use profiles of the three marriage duration categories of Protestant women are essentially similar.

Education differences in part reflect age differences, so comparisons between educational categories in table 50 must be made cautiously. While there are some variations among Catholics that tempt speculation, the differences between religious groups rather than within them are the pre-eminent facts exhibited in these figures.

[10] This percentage pertains to current users, not those who *ever* used the pill.

Table 48 Method Previously Used by Current Oral Contraceptors by Religion and Parity*

	Rhythm	*With-drawal*	*Dia-phragm*	*Vaginal Prepara-tions*	*Condom*	*I.U.D.*	*Other Methods*	*Total Per Cent*	*N*†
Roman Catholics									
All Parities	44.2	11.7	13.0	5.2	23.4	0.0	2.6	100.0	77
1–2 Parities	38.2	5.9	5.9	8.8	32.4	0.0	8.8	100.0	34
3+ Parities	47.6	16.7	19.0	2.4	9.5	0.0	4.8	100.0	42
Protestants									
All Parities	10.2	8.2	30.2	10.6	35.5	2.0	3.3	100.0	245
1–2 Parities	14.2	9.4	21.7	8.5	40.6	0.9	4.7	100.0	106
3+ Parities	7.9	6.3	39.7	12.7	27.8	3.2	2.4	100.0	126

**Excludes use "for medical purposes."*
†Sub-totals do not add to grand total because of item Non-Response.
Zero parity not shown.

Table 49 Method Last Used by Current Oral Contraceptors by Onset of Use and Religion

	Rhythm	*With-drawal*	*Dia-phragm*	*Vaginal Prepara-tions*	*Condom*	*I.U.D.*	*Other Methods*	*Total Per Cent*	*N**
Used Pill before 1965									
All	15.6	7.4	34.4	13.1	27.0	0.0	2.5	100.0	122
Roman Catholics	38.1	4.8	28.6	9.5	14.3	0.0	4.8	100.0	21
Protestant	10.9	5.4	37.0	14.1	31.5	0.0	1.1	100.0	92
Used Pill after 1965									
All	17.9	11.4	21.4	7.0	36.6	2.2	3.5	100.0	229
Roman Catholics	45.6	14.0	7.0	3.5	26.4	0.0	3.5	100.0	57
Protestants	9.9	9.9	26.3	8.6	38.2	3.2	3.9	100.0	152

**Sub-totals do not add to grand total because of item Non-Response.*

Fertility Rates and Adoption of Oral Contraception[11]

The rapid adoption of orals both as a new method and as a switch from other methods focuses attention on the reasons for adoption and the demographic implications of such a switch. While there has been considerable speculation concerning the impact of oral contraceptives on the recent decline in fertility rates there is little empirical evidence directly linking the two. One way of inferring something about the impact of orals is to compare the previous fertility of those who adopted orals with those who did not. In addition, we can examine whether those who took to orals early did so because they were experiencing higher fertility, by comparing them with those who adopted orals later.

User Status

Women in the survey were asked to look at a specially prepared calendar and state the months and years in which they took the pill. The women were considered to be confirmed pill users if they replied in the affirmative for at least three consecutive months of the year under consideration.[12]

There was very little oral usage before 1963. By the end of 1964, 207 women of the 691 who would eventually report usage for at least three consecutive months before the end of the series, were employing oral contraception. These women were classified as earlier adopters. By the end of 1965, 145 more began to use orals leaving 338 to begin use after December 1965. This latter category was classified as late adopters, thus providing a year's separation in time between early and late adopters. Together all 691 confirmed pill users formed a separate series as did all those who had never used oral contraceptives as of November 1967. Non-users numbered 729.

For each of the years 1959 through 1967, fertility rates were calculated for the different age and user categories. The means of these fertility rates are presented in table 51. It is evident that early users of orals previously had higher fertility than late users and that users in general have higher pre-use fertility than non-users. This pattern generally prevails across all age groups. As it now appears the pill must have contributed to lower fertility both because of the switching which occurred from less effective methods and because it was

[11] Analysis presented in this section was originally made by Don Lavis in his Master's thesis, "Ontario: The Pill and the Birth Rate, 1960–1967."

[12] This eliminated those who discontinued use shortly after adoption because of side effects or other reasons.

Table 50 Method Last Used by Current Oral Contraceptors by Religion, Duration of Marriage, and Education*

	Rhythm	*With-drawal*	*Dia-phragm*	*Vaginal Prepara-tions*	*Condom*	*I.U.D.*	*Other Methods*	*Total Per Cent*	*N*†
Roman Catholics									
Married 1954 or before	59.1	4.5	18.2	4.5	13.6	0.0	0.0	100.0	22
Married 1955–59	37.0	22.2	18.5	3.7	14.8	0.0	3.7	100.0	27
Married 1960 on	39.3	7.1	3.6	7.1	39.3	0.0	3.6	100.0	28
Protestants									
Married 1954 or before	9.7	3.9	36.9	10.7	32.0	2.9	3.9	100.0	103
Married 1955–59	9.0	9.0	34.6	9.0	34.6	1.3	2.5	100.0	78
Married 1960 on	12.1	13.6	13.6	12.1	40.9	1.5	6.1	100.0	66
Roman Catholics									
Less than grade 12	36.2	17.0	17.0	6.4	21.3	0.0	2.1	100.0	47
Grade 12 or more	50.0	2.9	5.9	2.9	23.6	0.0	14.7	100.0	34
Protestants									
Less than grade 12	10.5	7.4	27.4	11.1	37.0	2.2	4.4	100.0	135
Grade 12 or more	9.1	9.1	33.6	10.0	33.6	1.8	2.7	100.0	110

* *Excludes use "for medical purposes."*

† *Sub-totals do not add to grand total because of item Non-Response.*

Table 51 Mean Pre-Use Fertility Rates, per 100 (1959–1967), for Different Categories of Oral Users by Age

Comparison of Usage Categories	*Age* 20–24	25–29	30–34	35–39
Pill	31.4	30.4	24.6	16.4
vs.	*	*	*	*
Non-Pill	22.3	24.8	17.2	10.3
Early User	40.3	33.0	26.1	19.0
vs.	*			
Late User	26.3	27.4	26.3	13.5
Early User	40.3	33.0	26.1	19.0
vs.	*	*	*	*
Non-User	22.3	24.8	17.2	10.3
Late User	26.3	27.4	26.3	13.5
vs.			*	
Non-User	22.3	24.8	17.2	10.3

**Denotes statistically significant difference at the .05 level.*
Age group 40+ is omitted due to limited numbers.

Table 52 Future-Use Plans of Women Not Currently on the Pill, by Marriage-Duration Category

Future Use Plans	*Marriage Duration, Months* Under 72	72–107	108–143	144–179	180–227	228 or More	All Durations
Total							
Number	220	162	172	159	193	232	1138
Percentage	100.0	100.0	100.0	100.0	100.0	100.0	100.0
Will Use	33.7	26.5	26.2	13.2	16.1	11.6	21.1
Will Not Usc	51.8	59.3	63.9	79.9	74.1	83.2	68.9
Uncertain	14.5	14.2	9.9	6.9	9.8	5.2	10.0

adopted by those who previously had borne more children and were thus of demonstrated fecundity, fully capable of progressing to higher parities. There is an obvious implication here that pressure resulting from high fertility was instrumental to some degree in bringing about the adoption of a more efficient method of contraception.

Future Use of Oral Contraception

Earlier in this chapter, an examination of oral use trends by cohorts seemed to indicate that the rapid increase in the use of orals may be coming to an end and use in any cohort may be stabilized at a level well below 50 per cent. In this section we will examine future use plans of women not on the pill at the time of the interview.

The percentage of women not on the pill at the time of the interview, planning to use the pill in the future is inversely related to marriage duration (table 52). However, even among women of the shortest duration category (those married less than six years), only about a third say they plan to use the pill in the future. In all other duration categories a smaller fraction plans future use of the pill. Overall, about one in five women not now using the pill plan to do so in the future. Thus if we assume that all women now using orals continue to do so and that all women who say they plan to use orals in the future do so, use would rise to about 44 per cent of all women in the sample or about 52 per cent of fecund women. This in all likelihood is a high estimate of use since there are women currently on the pill who have indicated that they will decline future use. These estimates are hazardous on several counts, not the least being that both oral users and non-users may change their minds about future use.

Concern over the health hazard is, for all but the longest duration category, the major reported deterrent to oral contraceptive use (table 53). The positive relationship between sterility and marriage duration distorts the other percentages in table 53. By removing women reporting sterility[13] as the reason for future non-use a less marked inverse relationship between the percentage reporting "health hazard," and marriage duration results. As we have seen earlier (table 39) the use of orals as the sole method of contraception is most prevalent among couples married less than six years. It may be, therefore, that the data in table 53 relating to the health hazards and concern with side effects reflect the fact that those not on pills who have been married a relatively short time tend more towards hard-core resistance than is true of women who have been married longer. That is to say, couples who have been married recently and are looking for a method of contraception are attracted to orals unless they find them unacceptable. Couples married for a longer time and already accustomed to older methods are more prone to be satisfied with

[13] The proportion reporting sterility as a reason is an incomplete count of those currently sterile since some sterile women gave other reasons for not planning future use.

Table 53 Reasons Given against Future Use of Pill by Women Not Currently Using the Pill by Marriage-Duration Category

Reason Given	*Under 72*	*72–107*	*108–143*	*144–179*	*180–227*	*228 or more*	*All Durations*
	Marriage Duration, Months						
Total							
Number*	145	117	123	138	161	203	887
Percentage	100.0	100.0	100.0	100.0	100.0	100.0	100.0
Health Hazard	46.2	41.1	35.0	37.7	31.7	24.1	35.0
Side Effects	20.7	18.0	17.1	18.8	18.6	8.9	16.5
Present Method Satisfactory	11.7	8.5	14.6	10.2	21.7	17.3	14.5
Sterility	3.4	5.1	10.6	11.6	14.4	31.6	14.3
Religious Objections	9.0	14.5	11.4	10.1	8.7	10.3	10.4
Other, Including Combined Reasons	9.0	12.8	11.3	11.6	4.9	7.8	9.3

**Consists of women not using the pill who did not plan to use orals in the future or were uncertain.*

what they are using. This appears to be the case, for if we remove from consideration the couples who give sterility as their reason for non-use, we find that those married for the longest period are about twice as likely to find their present method satisfactory.

Few, if any, of the reasons given for planning to abstain from the use of orals can be considered "soft" in the sense of being easily dissipated. Indeed, reports in the mass media since the completion of the survey, relating to the health hazard of oral use may well decrease the precentage of women planning to use the pill, and increase the termination rates among current users.

Implications

For any duration category, the maximum proportion of women which could reasonably be found to be using orals even allowing for planned future use will be considerably less than unity. If fertility and sterility patterns retain in the near future their present configuration, the combined percentages of pregnant and sterile shown in table 54 will not, to any important extent, be at risk for pill usage. Furthermore, a proportion of women will not be using orals or any other method since they will be anticipating conception.

Table 55 shows the projected maximum percentage of oral use in each duration category under the assumptions that the percentage pregnant or sterile will remain constant as a nonrisk group and that the percentages switching to orals from each of the three current method categories (that is, "not using any method," "using other method(s)") noted in table 54 follow stated intentions.

The percentages who "intend to use" were derived by multiplying the numbers of women in each of the three contraceptive use categories of table 54 by the proportion stating they planned to use the pill in the future. The summation of the derived numbers was then taken as a percentage of the total women in each duration category. The percentage who intend to use or were uncertain was calculated in similar fashion, using the combined proportion stating they planned to use orals in future, or were uncertain. The figures are not intended as a prediction but merely to illustrate what under present conditions appear to be the upper limits of oral use. While not all women will use oral contraception, its use by over half of the women in their first twelve months of marriage would be a fact of great significance for future fertility. Other methods may replace orals to some extent, as for example voluntary sterilization or post-conception methods but it would be surprising indeed if methods less effective in avoiding births were to be adopted by these women.

Table 54 Pregnancy Risk Status and Contraceptive Status of Those at Risk by Marriage Duration

	Marriage Duration, Months						
Status	*Under 72*	*72–107*	*108–143*	*144–179*	*180–227*	*228 or more*	*All Durations*
Total							
Number	375	235	263	220	254	280	1627
Percentage	100.0	100.0	100.0	100.0	100.0	100.0	100.0
Pregnant or sterile	18.7	12.7	15.6	19.1	19.7	33.6	20.1
(Pregnant)	(14.4)	(7.2)	(3.4)	(1.8)	(0.4)	(0.4)	(5.3)
(Sterile)	(4.3)	(5.5)	(12.2)	(17.3)	(19.3)	(33.2)	(14.8)
At Risk	81.3	87.2	84.4	80.9	80.3	66.4	79.9
(Not using any method)	(20.3)	(21.7)	(19.8)	(16.4)	(18.9)	(21.8)	(19.9)
(Using orals)	(39.7)	(30.6)	(33.8)	(27.3)	(21.2)	(16.0)	(28.9)
(Using other method(s))	(21.3)	(34.9)	(30.8)	(37.2)	(40.2)	(28.6)	(31.3)

Figure 10 illustrates the extent to which increases in the use of orals can be expected under present fertility and sterility rates, and assuming the distribution of intentions regarding future use of oral contraceptives expressed by our sample.

Continuation Rates among Oral Users

The demographic impact of any contraceptive method depends not only on the use-effectiveness of the method but also on the length of time it is used uninterruptedly. Ever since orals first came into use, there have been many attempts to study the termination rates among oral users and the reasons for terminations. The purpose of this section is to analyse the pattern of terminations among oral pill users in our sample of women.[14]

Since orals have been available in Canada on a prescription basis only since 1961, and the number of women using them before then is very small, only the women who started using the pills on or after January 1962 are included in the analysis here. There were 732 such women. Further only the first segment of use by these women is considered for the construction of rates. This segment is the period of use from first use to first termination of use or to the time of survey when there has been no termination.

Table 55 Current and Projected Oral Use Rates by Marriage Duration *

Marriage Duration (Months)	*Current Users*	*Intend to Use***	*Intend to Use or Uncertain*
All	28.9	38.1	44.4
Under 72	39.7	49.6	55.7
72–107	30.6	44.2	54.5
108–143	33.8	45.6	51.7
144–179	27.3	32.1	37.7
180–227	21.2	29.9	36.6
228 or more	16.0	19.6	25.4

**Assumes no change in per cent pregnant or sterile and that future use of orals follows stated intention.*
***Includes current users of oral contraception.*

[14] See Appendix C for a technical presentation of the life table analysis of continuation rates.

That these data were collected through a sample survey rather than from a clinical study deserves comment. Firstly, the problem of follow-up loss does not arise in survey data as information is collected retrospectively. Secondly, retrospective data are subject to "recall lapse" despite efforts to overcome it. This survey employed the familiar device of a calendar with months indicated for a number of years. We asked the respondent to indicate the months of use. Besides the problem of recall lapse there is a technical hitch to this method since pill usage is related to menstrual cycles rather than calendar months. Thus, use over a cycle may be indicated as use in two adjacent months. On the average, therefore, it is possible for exposure time to be slightly overestimated to the extent of a half month. Our analysis of the significance of this factor on continuation rates suggests that it is not likely to be of much consequence.

Looking at overall continuation rates, it can be seen that about one-third of the first segments terminate by the end of the first year and about 47 per cent by the second year. At the end of four years the first segment continuation rate is only 32 per cent (table 56). Our results are very similar to those found in the United States in 1965 in a national sample survey by Westoff and Ryder.[15]

Terminations by Cause

The decrement rates for various causes by length of first segment are presented in table 57. These rates have been called net rates to distinguish them from the absolute rates calculated later in this section. The net rates are calculated by formulae which make allowance for the fact that if the loss rate is uniform, those who stop use in a given quarter are on the average exposed only half the time to the risk of pregnancy or other decrements.

Reasons given for discontinuation of oral pills were grouped into three categories: "planning pregnancy," "medical and health," and "other." Medical and health reasons include headache, nausea, spotting, and worry over threat to health. "Other" includes such varied reasons as "too expensive" and "could not remember to take the pills."

Medical and health reasons predominate in the first six months, accounting for over half the drop-outs, but become comparatively less important later. The pattern for other causes is less distinct suggesting the operation of random factors on contraceptive behaviour.

[15] Jones and Mauldin, "Use of Oral Contraceptives with Special Reference to Developing Countries."

Figure 10 Distribution of Women by Current Pregnancy or Sterility Status and the Remainder into Current and Prospective Users of Oral Contraceptives

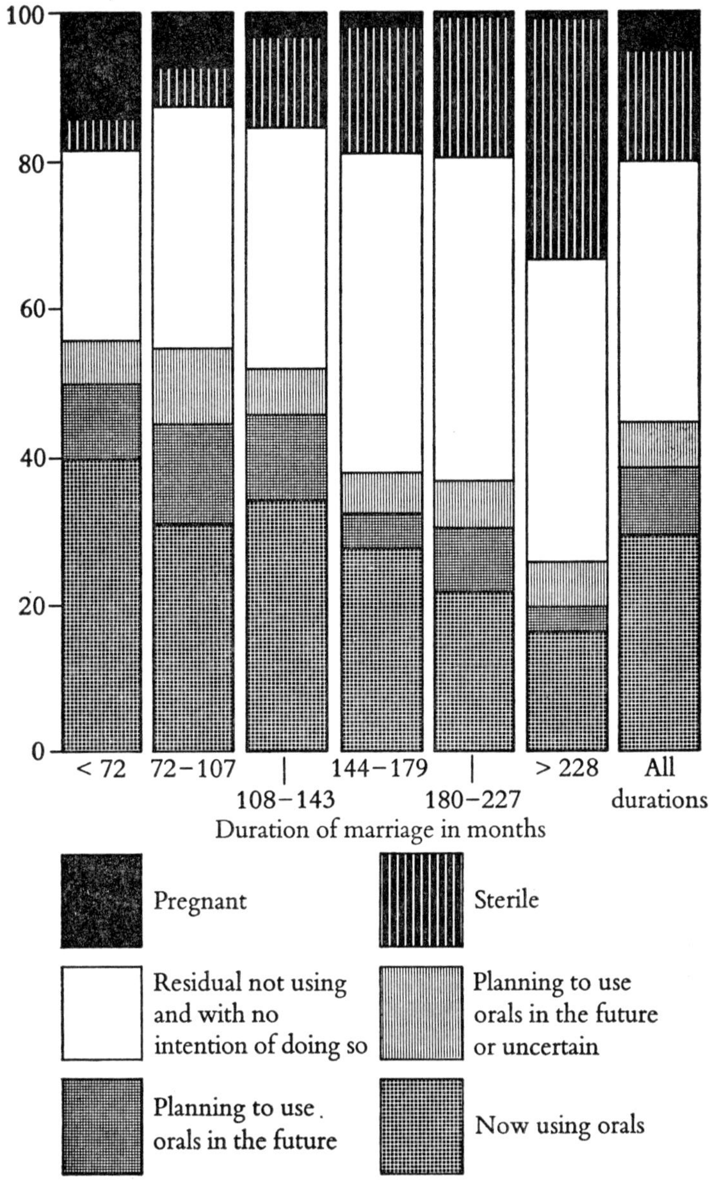

Discontinuation for pregnancy appears to become relatively unimportant between 16 and 24 months but has several apogees: after one half year of use, after two years of use, and after three years of use.

Table 56 Continuation Rates * for Oral Contraceptors

Months of Exposure	*Canadian Family Growth Study 1968*	*Westoff–Ryder U.S. 1965*
6	77	78
12	65	68
18	58	62
24	53	53
36	42	n.a.
48	32	n.a.

**First segment only; i.e., users who resume use after discontinuation not included.*

Absolute Rates of Decrement

The above stated net rates are not independent of each other. For comparative purposes it is probably more meaningful to look at the underlying absolute or true rates of decrement for each type of termination. These absolute rates are the rates that would be observed if other competing risks were not present. The absolute rate will always be slightly higher than net rates.

These absolute rates along with the corresponding continuation rates are presented in table 58. The patterns of discontinuation are virtually identical with those in table 57. It is clear from table 58 that medical and health reasons for discontinuation take the greatest toll of users.

As the single most commonly used measure in effectiveness studies is the continuation rate after specific durations, it will be of interest to look at the relationship between total continuation rates and the decomposed single decrement continuation rates. The merit of absolute rates of decrement is that, apart from giving true independent measures of decrement, the products of the single decrement continuation rates will be almost identical to total continuation rates.

In clinical studies where the number of women covered is large it may be possible to construct multiple decrement life tables separately for each cohort of women. However, in cross-section surveys where the sample size is usually small due to cost considerations, the multiple decrement life table is a useful device for synthesizing attrition data. It has the advantage of making use of varied pieces of experi-

Table 57 Net Decrement Rates by Cause of Termination and Length of Exposure

Months of Exposure	*Probability of Termination (Net Rates)* Plan Pregnancy	Medical, Health	Other	Total	*Cumulative Continuation Rate*
1–3	.0209	.0894	.0419	.1522	.8478
4–6	.0174	.0573	.0208	.0955	.7668
7–9	.0243	.0385	.0264	.0892	.6984
10–12	.0141	.0188	.0400	.0729	.6475
13–15	.0190	.0407	.0108	.0705	.6019
16–18	.0094	.0125	.0125	.0344	.5811
19–21	.0070	.0105	.0105	.0280	.5648
22–24	.0079	.0356	.0119	.0554	.5336
25–27	.0292	.0329	.0094	.0705	.4960
28–30	.0112	.0056	.0281	.0449	.4738
31–33	.0196	.0327	.0196	.0719	.4397
34–36	.0164	.0082	.0164	.0410	.4217
37–39	.0202	.0101	.0101	.0404	.4046
40–42	.0361	.0241	.0602	.1204	.3559
43–45	.0317	.0317	.0159	.0793	.3276
46–48	.0213	.0000	.0000	.0213	.3206
49+					

ence in order to derive statements about the probability of continuation or discontinuation of use specific for given durations. But as it blends the experience of different cohorts, there is no reason for the probabilities of a particular table to apply to populations other than the one for which the table was developed. We know that there are large differences between populations in the attrition experienced with similar contraceptive methods. In Taiwan, for example, oral discontinuation rates are reported to be very high. According to data from the 1968 follow-up survey in Taiwan, only 31 per cent of acceptors were still using orals after 12 months, including all segments of use.[16] The continuation rate for the present sample at 12 months was 65 per cent, for first segment use alone. Such disparities reflect many underlying differences in the age and parity of the samples, alternative methods available, general motivational levels, and other factors,

[16] Chen, Chang, Sun, and Gernada, "First Island Wide Pill Acceptor Follow-up Survey, 1968."

Table 58 Absolute Decrement Rates and Continuation Rates by Cause and Length of Exposure

	Absolute Decrement Rates			*Continuation Rates*			*Product of Columns*	*Total*
Months of Exposure	*Planning Pregnancy*	*Medical, Health*	*Others*	*Planning Pregnancy*	*Medical, Health*	*Others*	*(5) × (6) × (7)*	*Continuation Rate*
1–3	.0224	.0923	.0443	.9776	.9077	.9557	.8480	.8478
4–6	.0181	.0584	.0216	.9599	.8547	.9350	.7671	.7668
7–9	.0251	.0395	.0273	.9358	.8209	.9095	.6987	.6984
10–12	.0145	.0193	.0407	.9222	.8051	.8725	.6478	.6475
13–15	.0195	.0413	.0111	.9042	.7718	.8628	.6022	.6019
16–18	.0095	.0126	.0126	.8956	.7620	.8519	.5814	.5812
19–21	.0071	.0106	.0106	.8893	.7540	.8429	.5652	.5649
22–24	.0081	.0360	.0122	.8820	.7269	.8326	.5339	.5336
25–27	.0288	.0335	.0097	.8567	.7025	.8246	.4962	.4960
28–30	.0114	.0057	.0283	.8469	.6985	.8012	.4740	.4737
31–33	.0201	.0334	.0201	.8299	.6752	.7851	.4399	.4396
34–36	.0166	.0083	.0166	.8161	.6695	.7720	.4219	.4216
37–39	.0204	.0103	.0103	.7995	.6627	.7641	.4048	.4046
40–42	.0377	.0253	.0621	.7693	.6459	.7167	.3561	.3559
43–45	.0325	.0325	.0164	.7443	.6249	.7049	.3279	.3277
46–48	.0213	.0000	.0000	.7285	.6249	.7049	.3209	.3207
49+								

including possible differences in physical and psychological tolerance of the compound itself and its side effects.

It is of interest therefore to find that the continuation rates for the Canadian sample resemble closely those for the U.S. two years earlier. Differences in the composition of these two samples and the greater prevalence of use of orals by the time of the later study, apparently had little effect on the general pattern of attrition. This suggests the notion that, as with mortality tables, there may be families of decrement tables appropriate for particular types of populations. The idea obviously needs further investigation by examining attrition patterns by type of decrement for specified populations.

Continuation Rates by Religion and Education of Wife

Sample size limitations preclude construction of reliable continuation rates for subgroups. Nevertheless they are constructed for religious and educational categories in the hope that they may reveal existing patterns despite the problem of stability. These are presented in table 59. Continuation rates are slightly higher for Protestants than for Catholics. At the end of two years 59 per cent of the Protestant users were still on the pill compared to 49 per cent among the Catholics. Education seems to have little effect on continuation rates, the differences being minimal both at the end of one year and two years. As religion in our sample is correlated with the education of wife, it would have been more appropriate to look at continuation rates by religion of wife controlling for education. Such a refinement was not possible due to small numbers.

Medical Supervision of Oral Contraception

The long-run implications of using progestational compounds for contraception are not known. However, there seems little doubt that oral contraceptives are a cause of deep-vein thrombosis and embolism.[17] Certain other potentially serious effects are suspected though definitive evidence is generally lacking. Thus, there is reason for concern over the medical supervision of patients on oral contraceptives.

There are acknowledged problems in characterizing medical practice on the basis of the patient's retrospective reports although, of course, what the patient believes to be true is not without some significance in itself. Our assumption here is that these data probably

[17] *British Medical Journal*, "Oral Contraception and Thromboembolism."

give reasonably accurate aggregate descriptions of medical supervision in the case of oral contraceptives.

All women on orals at the time of the survey were asked among other things, the following questions: "For how many months was your last prescription for the pill?"; "When you first began taking the pill, did the doctor examine your breasts or give you an internal examination?"; "Did you have an internal examination the last time you had your prescription renewed?"; and "Did this examination include a 'Pap Smear' (Cancer Smear)?"

Table 59 Continuation Rates for Oral Contraceptors by Religion and Education of Wife *

	Number of Women	*Continuation Rate 12 Months*	*24 Months*	*36 Months*
Religion				
Protestant	498	70	59	46
Catholic	171	65	49	41
Others	63	55	45	34
Education				
Less than 8th grade	84	63	52	46
Grade 9–11	301	64	55	44
Grade 12–13	239	65	50	37
College	108	68	57	44
Total	732	65	53	41

**First segment use only; i.e., users who resumed use after discontinuation not included.*

Incidence of Initial Examinations

Of the 480 women using the pill at the time of the survey,[18] 83 per cent reported they had received an examination before receiving their first prescription while 17 per cent claimed no such examination was given.[19] Some proportion of this latter group may have been examined for other purposes a short time before beginning the use of orals. We have no information on this but it seems unlikely that many of those not examined are to be explained this way. Thus, allowing for sampling error, it would appear that from 14 to 20 per cent of women

[18] Women who had discontinued use of the pill were excluded to minimize recall bias.

[19] 95 per cent confidence limits on the observed percentage of 17 provide a range of 14.4 to 19.6 per cent.

received their first prescription for orals without examination of the type specified in this question.

Prescription Renewals and Physical Examination

The request by a patient for a prescription renewal provides an opportunity to make an examination and do a Papanicolaou Smear Test. The percentage of women reporting such examinations on last renewal is therefore of some interest, although not without problems of interpretation.

The population answering the last two questions was comprised of women currently on orals who had a prescription renewal. Of the 434 such women in the sample, 37 per cent denied having an internal examination when their prescription was last renewed. Since prescriptions are written for varying numbers of cycles and patients holding prescriptions for less than six cycles would not all receive examinations on last renewal, interpretation of this finding in relation to the standard is complex, unless an analysis is made in terms of prescription durations. The distribution of oral users by duration of current prescription is shown in table 60.

Table 60 Oral Users by Number of Cycles per Prescription

Number of Prescription Cycles	*Number of Current Users*	*Percentage*
One	92	19.2
Two–Three	68	14.2
Four–Five	7	1.5
Six	150	31.2
Seven–Eleven	11	2.3
Twelve	117	24.3
Thirteen or More	35	7.3
Total	480	100.0

About 35 per cent of women currently on orals have prescriptions for five or fewer cycles. If we assume, optimistically, that such women, on average, are examined every *second* renewal, we would expect about half of them to have had an examination at the last renewal. The percentage of this group receiving an examination on their last renewal was actually about 39 per cent (table 61).[20]

[20] The difference between 39 per cent and the expected value of 50 per cent is statistically significant at the .005 level. All differences commented on in the text are significant at P less than .05.

The percentage examined on last renewal increases with the duration of the prescription up to 12 cycles. Beyond that, rate of examination falls to 80 per cent. One view of this is that physicians who prescribe for long periods are also less meticulous than others about examining their patients. Alternatively, women receiving prescriptions for fewer cycles may present relatively more abnormalities and thus be examined more regularly.

Those who had received an examination on last renewal were asked if that examination included a "pap smear." About 89 per cent of 272 women[21] reported receiving a "pap smear" during their examination while 11 per cent said no such test was included.

Age of Patient and Probability of Examination

There is no overall relationship between age, as here classified, and probability of examination. When, as in table 62, we examine the probability of examination on last renewal, paying attention simultaneously to age and prescription duration, we also find that overall there is no statistically significant difference between the two broad age groups. The similarity within age groups in the proportions not examined by prescription duration suggests that prescription duration is not a factor in determining examination status and also that examination results may affect prescription duration.

Table 61 Percentage Examined by Prescription Duration

	Duration of Prescription in Cycles				
	1–5	*6–11*	*12*	*13 or More*	*Total*
Examined	39.1	62.4	92.3	80.0	62.7
Not Examined	60.9	37.6	7.7	20.0	37.3
Number of Cases	151	149	104	30	434

The pap smear test is evidently a very common feature of the examination. Overall, about 12 per cent of the women reported no such examination. When considered by age group the probability of receiving a pap smear shows no regular variation by age. As in table 62, the similarity in percentage distributions within age groups is more striking than the differences.

[21] Excludes "don't know."

Table 62 Percentage Not Receiving an Internal Examination at Last Renewal by Duration of Prescription and Age

Prescription Duration in Cycles	Less than 30 Years of Age		30 Years of Age or Older	
	Number	Not Examined	Number	Not Examined
One to five	52	63.5	99	59.6
Six	58	43.1	83	37.3
Seven or more	62	8.1	80	11.3
Total	172	36.6	262	36.8

The likelihood of a physical examination and pap smear at last renewal was looked at also in connection with the national background and education of the patient. The data indicate that women with less than 12 years of education were somewhat less likely to report an examination on their last renewal (30 per cent) than were women with more education (44 per cent). This finding is consistent with numerous illustrations from medical sociology of differential treatment by social-class background. One might argue that better educated women might be more likely to report an examination but this interpretation would seem to conflict with the finding of no difference in the reporting of pap smears. It is possible that with less educated women somewhat greater reliance is placed on the pap smear test alone. There were no differences, incidentally, in the frequency of either the examination of pap smear association with the patient's national background.

Summary

Aggregate time series of oral contraceptive use are difficult to interpret because they are based on different categories of women whose own patterns of oral use vary considerably. There are substantial differences by religion, education, and nativity in the use of oral contraception. Thus, separate time series were constructed and analysed for various categories of women.

Interpretation of time series of use is further complicated by changing marital duration distributions resulting from the time-segmented use of data collected at one point in time. Assembly of data from a cross-sectional survey with respect to age and marital status for a time prior to the survey date changes the composition of the sample by truncation of the age distribution and its upper end and by elimination of women whose eligibility for the sample was established because they first married after the earlier date. Because of this dilemma, duration specific use rates were calculated and time series were constructed for different marriage cohorts. These series seem to indicate that oral use may level off at about the same level for the various cohorts.

Past contraceptive practices of current oral users indicate that over three-quarters of the married women now using orals switched from another method—in over 70 per cent of these cases from relatively efficient methods, chiefly the condom and diaphragm. Women who gave up inefficient methods for orals and hence those for whom the gain in protection is greatest, are disproportionately Roman Catholics. This difference in the switching patterns of Protestants and Catholics holds for all parities, marriage duration, and educational groups.

About two-thirds of present oral users began to use them for the first time after January 1965. Catholic women lagged slightly behind Protestant women in the adoption of orals but the similarity in response to the introduction of this new method is as notable as the difference.

There is no appreciable difference in switching patterns among Protestants who were early adopters and those who were late adopters. Among Catholics there is a difference—somewhat more of the late adopters have come over from inefficient methods than was true of early adopters. While it is tempting to see in this some evidence that orals are becoming more acceptable to Catholics, other interpretations cannot be eliminated.

A comparison of pre-use fertility rates of pill users with non-pill users shows that pill users had higher fertility rates than non-pill users before switching to the pill. Also those who adopted the pill early had higher fertility than those who adopted late. It would thus appear that the pill must have contributed to lower fertility both because of the switching from less effective methods and because it was adopted by those who had a higher demonstrated fertility.

A look at continuation rates indicates that about one-third of first segments of use terminate by the end of the first year and about 47 per cent by the second year. At the end of four years the continuation rate is only 32 per cent. Medical and health reasons predominate in the first six months, accounting for over half the drop-outs, but becoming comparatively less important later.

Data on medical supervision of oral use obtained from the respondents reveal some minor lapses from what might be regarded as ideal practice. Some prescriptions are given for periods of more than a year thus forfeiting an opportunity for surveillance. Despite the increased medical risks associated with age, there is no evidence that age has much influence on examination protocol. Put more positively, we might say that the frequency of internal examination and administration of the pap smear test are as conscientiously performed with young as with older patients. Examinations of women of below average education is somewhat less thorough in some cases and evidence of greater caution with older users is lacking. Most oral users, however, appear to be well supervised.

6

Attitudes towards Abortion[1]

Abortion is rapidly becoming an important public issue in Canada. Its legal, moral, and political implications are widely debated, and many organizations are pressing for liberalization of old abortion laws. In June 1969, the Canadian Parliament passed a controversial series of amendments to the Criminal Code of Canada, which approved abortions where the mother's health was seriously endangered by the continuation of a pregnancy. Since then, some increase in therapeutic abortions has been observed in certain communities.[2] However, the impact of the amendments themselves on the incidence has been questioned.[3] Recently, the Royal Commission on the Status of Women recommended strongly that abortions be permitted by a qualified medical practitioner solely on the request of any woman who has been pregnant for 12 weeks or less or at the request of a woman pregnant for more than 12 weeks if the doctor is convinced that the continuation of the pregnancy would endanger the physical or mental health of the woman, or if there is a substantial risk that if the child were born, it would be greatly handicapped either mentally or physically.[4] In the light of the above recommendations and the general

[1] A slightly revised version of this chapter was published earlier. See T. R. Balakrishnan *et al.*, "Attitudes Toward Abortion of Married Women in Metropolitan Toronto."

[2] Boyce and Osborn, "Therapeutic Abortion in a Canadian City."

[3] Veevers, "The Liberalization of the Canadian Abortion Laws."

[4] Government of Canada, *Report of the Royal Commission on the Status of Women in Canada*, pp. 281-87.

change in social attitudes, further legislation can be expected in the near future.

It will be especially appropriate to ascertain at this stage the attitudes of women directly affected by these laws. While there have been a limited number of studies in the United States, they have been practically non-existent in Canada.[5] In this chapter we shall analyse the responses of our sample of married women to a series of questions on abortion.

Our interest in abortion also arises from its possible demographic impact in the next few years. Countries which have liberalized abortion have all experienced sudden rapid decline in birth rates. Will the decline in birth rates in the United States and Canada be accelerated by liberalization of abortion laws? Will abortion be used as a means of birth control, or will it primarily be used as a means of removing accidental pregnancy where a birth-control method has failed? In the latter case, what proportion of accidentally pregnant women is likely to seek abortion?

A number of questions were asked about the respondents' approval of abortion under different situations. The distribution of responses to these questions is presented in table 63.

The responses reveal three patterns. Women overwhelmingly approved abortion if mother's health is endangered, if she is mentally ill or raped, and if there is a question of deformity of the newborn. They were somewhat undecided on situations of severe emotional or economic problems and were generally opposed if the grounds were that serious marriage difficulties might ensue, that the woman was not married, or that a couple simply did not want any more children.

Common to the first four situations described in table 63 is a dire consequence combined with a presumed non-volitional aspect. Circumstances beyond the woman's control are responsible for the unfortunate situation in which she finds herself. "More to be pitied than censured" as the old song had it.

Situations 5 and 6 involve serious consequences and from half to two-thirds of the respondents would favour abortion to avoid them. Nevertheless there is significantly less agreement that these situations constitute grounds for abortion perhaps because they see "emotional problems" and "economic hardship" as matters with which one can and should cope rather than attempt to escape. As the volitional

[5] Rossi, "Public Views on Abortion." Kantner and Allingham, "American Attitudes on Population Policy: Recent Trends." Westoff, Moore, and Ryder, "The Structure of Attitudes Towards Abortion." Ryder and Westoff, *Reproduction in the United States, 1965*, Chapter 10.

component increases disapproval increases sharply to the extent that when nothing other than the couples' desires are involved (situation 9), two-thirds express disapproval with very few taking an equivocal position.

Another way of looking at the responses in table 63 is to cumulate the number of positive responses in order to see what percentage endorse abortion under any or all of the nine situations we have described, what proportion approve in eight out of nine, seven out of nine, and so on down to the percentage that is opposed under any conditions. From the cumulative distribution by number of positive responses (below) it is revealed that 92 per cent approve of abortion for at least one reason—in most cases this is to save the mother's life, the only reason recognized as the basis for a legal abortion in Canada at the time of the survey.[6]

Number of Positive Responses	*Cumulative Distribution*
0	100
1	92
2	87
3	80
4	72
5	61
6	48
7	36
8	26
9	15

However, up to five reasons are accepted by 61 per cent of our respondents, indicating that at least among Toronto couples, public sentiment is more liberal than the law. The reasons accepted by the majority include psychiatric and emotional problems resulting from an additional child, the reasons which have formed the basis of very liberal abortion policies in other countries.

[6] No question was asked about changing the Canadian law. The figure of 87 per cent was derived from the number of respondents supporting more than one indication for abortion not permitted by law at the time. Because the attitude index is not perfectly scaleable the response patterns do not provide a precise indication of which items have been accepted or rejected. The degree of scaleability is, however, high enough to support the general validity of the interpretation we are making here.

Table 63 Percentage Distribution of Responses to Attitudes towards Abortion in Different Situations

Situation	*Yes*	*No*	*Unsure**
1. Having a child would endanger mother's life	87	8	5
2. Mother mentally ill or retarded	76	15	9
3. There is a strong chance of a deformed or mentally handicapped child	76	16	8
4. Pregnancy due to rape	75	16	9
5. Mother would experience severe psychiatric and emotional problems if not aborted	67	20	13
6. Having another child would mean extreme economic hardships for the couple	50	43	7
7. Serious marriage difficulties likely to result in divorce	31	56	13
8. Unmarried and does not wish to marry the father	30	56	14
9. Couple could afford another child but felt strongly that they did not want one	28	68	4

**Unsure includes a very small number of non-responses. Non-responses are less than one per cent for all questions.*

Abortion-on-demand which is indicated by situation 9 is endorsed by 28 per cent of the respondents. In the cumulative distribution, however, we see that only 15 per cent endorse all nine reasons which means that some who take what is presumably the most liberal position—abortion-on-demand—nevertheless have reservations about approving abortion in certain circumstances. Besides demonstrating that people are not always consistent in their views, it is possible that some of the situations as described were interpreted with greater than average discrimination. For example, one might agree that if a "couple," a term which suggests marriage, is strongly adverse to having "another child," suggesting they have fulfilled some of their reproductive obligations, they should not be forced to, but be allowed an abortion. Some persons who feel that way about a married couple may, however, not extend the same latitude to an unmarried woman (situation 8); or feel that having a child might "save a marriage" (situation 7); or fail to believe that another child could result in "extreme economic hardship"; etc.

At the other end of the scale, we find that only eight per cent (100–92) of our respondents are opposed to abortion for any reason whatsoever. This coincides as one would expect with the eight per cent who say they would not approve of an abortion even if the mother's life was endangered (table 63).

These responses are quite similar to those that have been elicited to similar questions in recent national surveys in the United States.[7] This is true despite differences between samples in religious composition, nativity, and other characteristics.

Overall the attitudes expressed by our respondents lie somewhere between those of the Roman Catholic affiliated organizations opposed to reform of present laws and those of Unitarian and Jewish organizations advocating a very liberal position towards abortion.

A reminder that attitudes are only a guide to behaviour is seen in the responses to the following question: "If you should accidentally become pregnant and already had all the children you want, do you think you might consider having an abortion to terminate the pregnancy if abortion for this reason were legal in Canada?"

Only 18 per cent responded in the affirmative and yet 38 per cent had approved abortion in this instance in principle (table 63). For non-Catholics the comparable figures were 22 and 35 per cent; for Catholics 7 and 13 per cent. This apparent inconsistency between an

[7] Jones and Westoff, "Attitudes Toward Abortion in the United States in 1970 and the Trend Since 1965."

attitude towards abortion and one's own readiness to act suggests the operation of intervening considerations such as loyalty to religious precepts or fear of the operation.

Measurement of Attitude towards Abortion

An index measuring the attitude towards abortion was developed using the responses to the nine questions in table 63. This index is the sum of the positive responses and thus can vary from 0 to 9 for any respondent. Thus if a woman expresses approval of abortion in six of the nine situations presented, her score will be 6. The mean abortion attitude score for all women was 5.19 with a standard deviation of 2.78. Construction of the index by a simple addition implies equal weight for all the questions. The higher the score for a respondent the more liberal is her attitude towards abortion.

Fertility Behaviour, Family Planning Practices, and Attitudes towards Abortion

The few studies on attitudes towards abortion conducted in North America all show that attitudes towards abortion are closely related to a person's religious beliefs, level of education, income, and so on.[8] But how far they are a function of a woman's situational factors—such as the number of children desired or expected, accidental pregnancy history, and contraceptive practice—are less often explored. However, Westoff, Moore, and Ryder did find in their 1965 national sample of United States women an inverse relation between number of children expected and liberal attitudes towards abortion.[9]

Examining first the influence of family size on the attitudes towards abortion (table 64) we observe that the general pattern is towards a less liberal attitude as family size increases. For both Catholics and non-Catholics there is an inverse relation between number of children (desired, expected, or actual) and liberality of attitude towards abortion after two children. However, women with no children or one child are less liberal than average. It is possible that these women are not immediately concerned with controlling their family size because they are either too young, just starting their families, or have problems of sterility or subfecundity.

8 Westoff, Moore, and Ryder, "Structure of Attitudes Towards Abortion," pp. 14-16.

9 Westoff, Moore, and Ryder, "Structure of Attitudes Towards Abortion," p. 25.

The converse situation would involve women who had failed in planning their families. Thus, those women who had accidental pregnancies resulting in either unwanted children or children at an unwanted time might be more liberal towards abortion. To test this hypothesis, all the women in the sample were classified according to whether their last pregnancy was unwanted in terms of number and spacing. The results are presented in table 65. Both among Catholics and non-Catholics, women whose last pregnancy was unwanted were more liberal towards abortion. A spacing failure does not affect responses as much as a number failure. Consistent with these findings is that 33 per cent of the women whose last pregnancy was unwanted said that they would obtain an abortion next time if they became pregnant and if it were legally available to them, as against 14 per cent of women whose last pregnancy was not accidental. Thus, past success or failure in family planning conditions attitudes towards abortion.

A related question is the relationship between contraceptive practice and attitudes towards abortion. An analysis of the relation between current contraceptive practice and attitudes towards abortion (table 66) shows the most liberal women to be those who were currently using mechanical methods (condom and diaphragm). Next in order of liberality of attitude were women on pills and I.U.D.; on chemicals and other methods and rhythm. Not surprisingly the greatest difference in attitude between Catholics and non-Catholics is found for women who were not using any method or using rhythm. Women who are on more effective methods are evidently more concerned about control of the family size and more prone to include abortion among the acceptable modes of control. Favourable attitudes towards abortion also are more likely among the less religious, the better educated, those with higher incomes, and those who were born in large cities (table 67). The less favourable attitudes of oral and I.U.D. users compared to those using mechanical methods may have something to do with age and parity or, especially in the case of Catholics, may reflect the moral ambiguity associated with orals during the period.

Socio-Economic Characteristics and Attitudes towards Abortion

Family size and contraception are at best intervening variables conditioned by socio-economic background, religious beliefs, and the values and norms of particular social milieux. The greatest differences

Table 64 Mean Abortion Attitude Score by Religion and Family Size Variables

Number of Children	*Catholic*	*Non-Catholic*	*Total*	*Number of Women*
Desired				
0 or 1	3.33	6.93	6.08	38
2	4.08	6.05	5.60	539
3	3.69	6.05	5.37	473
4	3.24	5.91	4.99	417
5	2.48	5.23	3.89	43
6 or more	2.03	5.03	3.57	68
Expected				
0 or 1	2.86	6.44	5.64	169
2	4.11	6.02	5.53	518
3	3.71	6.01	5.41	450
4	3.12	5.89	4.82	265
5	3.29	5.67	4.60	78
6 or more	1.85	5.67	4.14	65
Actual				
0 or 1	3.26	5.76	5.11	505
2	3.83	6.17	5.51	507
3	3.41	5.98	5.18	330
4	2.92	6.36	5.03	165
5	2.93	5.55	4.39	68
6 or more	2.15	5.96	4.34	47
Total*	3.35	5.93	5.19	1626

**The total number of women in this and other tables might not add to 1626 due to non-response.*

Table 65 Mean Abortion Attitude Score by Planning Status of Last Pregnancy

Last Pregnancy Status	*Catholic*	*Non-Catholic*	*Total*	*Number of Women*
Number failure	4.13	6.33	5.74	233
Spacing failure	3.72	5.90	5.10	212
All others	3.13	5.93	5.10	1181
Total	3.35	5.93	5.19	1626

Table 66 Abortion Attitude Score by Religion and Current Method of Contraception Used *

Method of Contraception	*Catholic*	*Non-Catholic*	*Total*	*N*
Condom and Diaphragm	5.37	6.26	6.13	285
Oral Pills and I.U.D.	3.91	6.10	5.62	523
Chemical and Other	3.71	5.81	5.06	126
Rhythm	2.58	5.11	3.62	88
None, at Risk	2.87	5.58	4.36	341
None, Not at Risk	2.88	6.03	5.00	263
Total	3.35	5.93	5.19	1626

* *When more than one method was used, only the most effective method was counted.*

Table 67 Abortion Attitude Score by Socio-Economic Characteristics

Socio-Economic Characteristics	*Mean Abortion Score*	*Number of Women*
Religion		
Catholic	3.36	492
Protestant	5.97	974
Jewish	6.89	62
Others	5.49	96
Religiosity (Church Attendance)		
Don't attend	6.02	551
Rarely attend	5.23	482
Less than 5 times a month	4.15	394
5 or more times a month	3.57	196
Education		
8 years of schooling or less	3.76	355
9 to 11 years of school	5.29	603
12 years of school	5.43	397
At least some university*	5.84	263

Table 67 (Continued)

Socio-Economic Characteristics	*Mean Abortion Score*	*Number of Women*
Husband's Annual Income		
Less than $5,000	3.60	208
$5,000 to $5,999	4.84	274
$6,000 to $7,999	5.14	393
$8,000 to $9,999	5.79	227
$10,000 or more	6.24	360
Size of Birthplace		
Less than 5,000 population	4.46	387
5,000 to 49,999	4.73	396
50,000 to 499,999	5.43	232
500,000 or more	5.87	606
Total	5.19	1626

**At least some university includes 150 women who had completed grade 13 which is equivalent to first year of college in provinces outside Ontario.*

in abortion attitude are those associated with religious affiliation (table 67). The mean abortion index for Catholics was 3.36 compared to 5.97 for Protestants and 6.89 for Jews. The next important factor was religiosity as measured by church attendance. Women who don't attend church have a mean abortion index of 6.02 compared to 3.57 for those who attend church five or more times a month. Education and income are both positively related to liberality of attitudes. Since education and income are highly correlated, this consistency is to be expected. The wife's rural–urban background as measured by the size of her birthplace was also positively related to her attitudes towards abortion. The greatest difference falls at communities above and below 50,000 population.

Summary

The preceding analysis suggests that socio-economic characteristics are much more important in shaping a woman's attitudes towards abortion than situational variables such as having an accidental pregnancy, method of contraception, or desired number of children. Among the socio-economic variables, religion and religiosity are predominant. Our study seems to indicate that a decline in religious values and beliefs more than anything else would contribute towards liberalizing attitudes towards abortion.

7

An Overview

This study of family formation in a Canadian metropolis was undertaken in the hope that it would assist in understanding past fertility trends and might also point to the possible future course of fertility. As our sample is restricted to Metropolitan Toronto, generalizations to Canadian society as a whole are not permissible. In this final section we will stress the highlights of our findings and some of their implications.

The women in our sample share many common values about the size of the ideal family. Almost all consider the ideal Canadian family of average means to consist of two to four children with three as the most common value. Their own personal desires match these ideals closely. However, their actual fertility performance to the time of the survey when taken together with the number of additional children expected reveals that the average woman may fall short of achieving her family-size desires. To some degree this is the result of sterility and subfecundity.

But there is also a substantial degree of excess fertility as measured by the percentage reporting that their last child was unwanted in spite of a high level of contraceptive use. Such a level of excess fertility, which is just under 15 per cent for all couples and rises to almost 50 per cent for those who have more than four children indicates that the birth control that is practised is often ineffective. However, the amount of excess fertility indexed by whether or not the last child was wanted may be an underestimation. The question ignores earlier births that may have been unwanted and does not pick up those which were in fact unwanted but which the respondent could not bring herself to so describe. The policy implications of this fact for governmental and other agencies involved in widening family-planning services in Canada is clear. There is a job to do in aiding couples to reach the family size they desire, which in some cases will involve finding a solution to the problem of excess fertility and in others overcoming the problem of insufficient fertility. The matching of performance to desires is much more the problem than is the reduction or increase in overall fertility.

Toronto couples express relatively low values with respect to the ideal, desired, and expected number of children. The suggested trend towards smaller families appears to be at least partially borne out by the declining birth rates of the last few years. However, it is difficult to separate a change in fertility values from the effect of increased contraceptive effectiveness which puts family-size desires more realistically within reach. The rapid adoption of oral contraception in the recent past is most dramatic. From the analysis of the extent of oral pill use, however, it is our conclusion that the impact of orals alone cannot explain the fertility decline. A basic change towards lower family-size norms seems to be taking place in the population we have studied and, we would surmise, in the rest of Canada as well.

Fertility differentials by socio-economic characteristics generally follow patterns found in similar surveys in other developed countries. Religion, education, and wife's labour force status are predominant factors in fertility behaviour. Income and occupation have a U-shaped relationship, rather than the inverse relationship often encountered. That is, fertility is highest at the extremes of income and occupation; lowest in the middle. Differences in fertility by religion are the expected ones, with Catholics exhibiting relatively high fertility, Protestants and other groups, relatively low fertility. In contrast to the findings from certain other studies we find that religiosity, as measured by church attendance, and nativity behave differently than expected. Religiosity is positively related to fertility even among Protestants whereas previous findings would have led us to expect this only among Catholics. Foreign-born women have lower fertility, both actual and expected, than native-born women. They differ also with respect to family planning practices but not as expected: despite lower fertility, foreign-born women appear to be less inclined towards the use of contraception. A large proportion of foreign-born residents of Toronto are recent immigrants. It is possible that with increased time in Canada, family-size norms prevalent among native-born Canadians are assimilated by the immigrant women. Lack of adequate number of cases precluded analysis of fertility by date of immigration and age at immigration. It may be that the fact of immigration is less important than the degree of assimilation. If this is valid, young foreign-born women may complete their reproductive careers with about the same number of children as native-born women have had. The differences would be in the timing of births. On the other hand the family-size norm is a flexible one specifying merely that two to four children are expected in the normal case. Assimilation, therefore, even if it occurs does not exact great precision in reproductive performance and thus the differences observed here by nativity might well persist.

By far the highest degree of association is observed between the wife's employment patterns and fertility. Granted that it is difficult to establish a cause–effect relationship, the high correlation nevertheless suggests that the low fertility norms should be consolidated by the high levels of female employment which have been established in Canadian society. Although the upper limit of labour force participation for women is difficult to predict some further increase is predictable. Whether this leads to even lower fertility or merely more unwanted fertility depends on how effectively the new recruits to the labour force practise birth control.

Canadian women are overwhelmingly in favour of birth control and practise it widely. About two-thirds were using birth control at the time of the survey and as many as 86 per cent had used a method at some time. Even among the recently married and still childless, use was high, indicating planning for spacing as well as for number. The nature of contraception over the last decade has drastically changed with the advent of oral contraception. By the time of the survey oral contraception had become the most popular method with nearly half of all those using contraception using orals. However, there is considerable variation in oral use by age. It is very popular with the young, recently married women whose use rates are as high as 70 per cent. Among older women use rates are much lower. A time series analysis by cohorts shows that use rates have a tendency to level off after a few years. Because orals are a recent innovation, it is difficult to predict future use patterns, especially as this involves the balance between new acceptances and discontinuations. A study of continuation rates shows that in this population there is a fair rate of termination for a broadly defined set of health reasons.

It is surprising that oral pill use among Catholics who use contraception is not much lower than among Protestants. Moreover, those

Catholics who use the pill have shifted to it primarily from rhythm and other relatively inefficient methods. Thus increased oral use should have effected a disproportionate reduction in Catholic fertility. Among the Protestants on the other hand most oral pill users switched from other efficient methods such as the condom and the diaphragm and hence the impact on fertility is likely to be less than among Catholics. An investigation of past fertility rates of oral users shows that those who adopt orals tend to be of above average fertility. Thus while the future impact of oral use cannot be measured precisely, all indications are that orals will have a substantial and perhaps differential effect on fertility trends at least in the near future. The main difference overall between Catholics and Protestants is the prevalence of use: Catholics are about equally divided between current users and non-users; nearly 70 per cent of Protestants are current users. The potential for future change to more effective fertility regulation is clearly greatest among Catholics.

Attitudes towards abortion are more liberal than the law now on the books. The relatively tolerant attitudes towards abortion observed in this population adumbrate the subsequent movements towards liberalization which culminated in a relaxation of the laws themselves. Recent statistics show that legal therapeutic abortions in Canada have skyrocketed since the law was changed. A detailed analysis of abortion attitudes in our sample shows that attitudes are still basically determined by religious beliefs and to a lesser extent by other socio-economic characteristics. Personal experience of an unwanted birth also contributes towards a more liberal attitude towards abortion.

Implications

It is apparent from this study that there are wide differences among various groups with respect to their fertility, both actual and desired. For the population of Toronto we have perhaps thrown some light on the nature of these differences but have been able to go only a relatively short way towards explaining them. The same is true of the differences observed with respect to attitudes towards contraception and abortion and the practice of birth control. A better understanding of these differences, especially of the factors that give rise to them, is a necessary basis for any policy or program that would attempt to deal with them. It is also a matter of some scientific priority. To achieve this degree of understanding an investigation that goes beyond the limits of the size and locale of the present one is needed.

The uses of such an inquiry are not exhausted by reference to its value for programs of fertility regulation or its academic interest. Basic to planning in many sectors of society is a reasonable set of population projections. The greatest source of error in projecting population comes in the assumed course of fertility. No single study can be expected to solve the perplexing issues with which the projectionist has to contend but a beginning should be made on a national scale and with a sample large enough to trace out relationships with an acceptable degree of assurance as to the statistical reliability of the results. We trust that the present study will facilitate such an undertaking by identifying areas of ignorance by suggesting certain hypotheses and by passing on the hard lessons which make any study that bothers to learn from its predecessors, better than that which went before.

We have noted that the process of family formation is an imperfect one. For a very considerable proportion of married women, their expected reproductive reach exceeds their grasp. More poignantly perhaps, many women have more children than they want. The significance of this latter problem does not end with the acknowledgement of excess fertility but extends in subtle ways to the affectional tone of family life and works its way out into the personalities of succeeding generations. It may be no mere coincidence that recognition in the scientific literature of the extent of unwanted childbirth emerges at about the same time as concern for battered children, dyslexia, and other indications of family malfunctioning. We are not suggesting any simplistic causal formulations but merely wish to call attention to the need to know more about what makes for quantitative success in family building because of its possible implications for the quality of family life. Often overlooked is the obvious fact that unwanted children result not only from imperfect regulation but also from shrinking family size norms. As the margin for error is reduced the demand for more effective methods of control is intensified; and those who exceed the new limits feel the effect of their error more keenly. In analysing the phenomenon of excess fertility in this study we have isolated certain correlates but again because of the inherent limitations of our data have had to end the analysis before curiosity was satisfied.

The possibility is suggested by our data that except possibly for Catholic couples, the market for oral contraception may soon be fairly well saturated at a level that would still leave a sizeable demand for other contraceptive methods. With the rather high rate of discontinuation among the users of oral contraception, this implies the need for additional contraceptive methods of equal effectiveness if the efficiency of the family formation process is to be further enhanced. Alternatively, there might be profit in intensive studies of contraceptive failure since the present armamentarium of methods provides a high degree of effectiveness in fertility planning provided the necessary motivation and discipline exist.

As we have seen the attitudes towards abortion expressed by the respondents in this study are fully consonant with the recent liberalization of the statutes. There are very few women who appear to be completely opposed to abortion under any circumstances. At the same time only a minority endorses the idea of abortion-on-demand. There are pronounced differences on this question among subgroups of the population and while our analysis has identified some of these differences many questions remain. Especially unexpected are the attitudes of young women which imply a relative lack of support for a liberal abortion policy. A larger study of broader compass could and should pursue this problem to a more satisfactory level of explanation. With abortion becoming more common and with the development of indirect techniques for measuring its prevalence, it would be desirable to study the prevalence of abortion, ideally among subgroups of the population, as well as attitudes towards it.

In our view the next step should be to explore these questions over the entire spectrum of cultural differences that are represented in Canada. To a considerable extent, policy regarding population problems will be federal policy and our knowledge of the dynamics of population should therefore be national in scope. Isolated, ad hoc surveys, while suggestive, can never be more than that. This study has made it evident that attitudes and behaviour with respect to fertility are changing rapidly, that the reproductive lives of many couples fall short of what they would have preferred, and finally that there appear to be certain distinctive features to Canadian fertility. The time is overdue for an investigation commensurate with the scientific and practical importance of the questions involved. We offer this book as a first step in that direction.

Appendix A

Questionnaire

CONFIDENTIAL

UNIVERSITY OF WESTERN ONTARIO
LONDON CANADA
Canadian Family Growth Study

1. Have you ever had any children?
   1 Yes
   2 No
2. IF YES: How many live born children have you had?
   Number ______________

	Day	*Month*	*Year*
3. What was your date of birth?			
4. What was your husband's date of birth?			
5. And your marriage date?			

6. Have you or your husband ever been married before?
   1 Yes
   2 No

   IF "YES" FOR EITHER CONCLUDE INTERVIEW

7. In what country were you and your husband born?

Wife	*Husband*	
1	1	Canada
2	2	U.K.
3	3	Italy
4	4	Germany
5	5	Netherlands
		Other (specify) ____________

8. IF OTHER THAN CANADA ASK: In what year did you/your husband come to Canada?

	Wife	*Husband*
Year of arrival	____	____
If "DON'T KNOW" check	☐	☐

9. What language did you/your husband first learn to speak as a child?

Wife	*Husband*	
1	1	English
2	2	French
3	3	Italian
4	4	German
5	5	Dutch
6	6	Greek
7	7	Polish
8	8	Russian
		Other (specify) ____________

10. IF FIRST LANGUAGE NOT ENGLISH ASK:
Can you/your husband *speak* that language fluently now?

Wife	*Husband*	
1	1	Yes
2	2	No

11. IF "NO" (OR HESITANT) ASK: Can you/your husband understand others that speak it?

1	1	Yes
2	2	No

12. (a) Is a language other than English ever spoken in the home?
    1 No (Skip to Q. 13)
    2 Yes

12. (b) By whom? To what extent?

READ FIRST 3 BELOW	(1) Older Parent(s)	(2) Husband & Wife	(3) Couple's Children	(4) Other Situation	DESCRIBE BELOW
Frequently	1	1	1	1	
Sometimes	2	2	2	2	
Never	3	3	3	3	
Does Not Apply	0	0	0	0	
Name of Language					

13. (a) Have you/your husband always lived in Metropolitan Toronto?

Wife	*Husband*	
1	1	Yes
2	2	No

(IF BOTH "YES" SKIP TO Q. 14)

(b) How long have you/your husband lived here?

Wife	*Husband*	
1	1	Less than 1 year
2	2	1–2 years
3	3	3–5 years
4	4	6–10 years
5	5	11–20 years
6	6	21–30 years
7	7	Over 30 years
0	0	Don't know, won't say

14. How large was the community where you/your husband was born?

Wife	*Husband*	
1	1	On a farm
2	2	Village (less than 5,000)
3	3	Small town (5–19 thousand)
4	4	Small city (20–49 thousand)
5	5	Medium city (50–99 thousand)
6	6	Large city (100–499 thousand)
7	7	Metropolis (over 500 thousand)
0	0	Don't know; don't remember; won't say

15. How large was the community where you/your husband lived mostly when your were 8–13 years old?

1	1	On a farm
2	2	Village (less than 5,000)

3	3	Small town (5–19 thousand)
4	4	Small city (20–49 thousand)
5	5	Medium city (50–99 thousand)
6	6	Large city (100–499 thousand)
7	7	Metropolis (over 500 thousand)
0	0	Don't know; don't remember; won't say

16. During the years when you were 8–13 how much, if at all, did your mother work outside of the home?
    1 Usually, full time
    2 Usually, part time
    3 Some of the time at a full time job
    4 Some of the time at a part time job
    5 Seldom
    6 Never
    0 Don't remember, won't say

17. Were your parents living together continually during that time?
    1 Yes
    No (IF "NO" ASK WHY AND CIRCLE BELOW)
    2 Divorced or separated
    3 Mother deceased
    4 Father deceased
    5 Both deceased
    6 Father overseas
    0 Don't remember, won't say
    7 Other

18. With whom did you mostly live then?
    (i.e. when you were 8–13)
    1 Parents
    2 Mother only
    3 Father only
    4 Mother and Father at separate times
    5 Relatives
    6 Other
    0 Don't remember, won't say

19. When you were 14–18 years old with whom did you mostly live?
    1 Parents
    2 Mother only
    3 Father only
    4 Mother and Father at separate times
    5 Relatives

6 Other
0 Don't remember, won't say

20. (a) Some people have very definite ideas about the number of children in an ideal-sized family. Others have not given much thought to it. In your case, if you have a definite opinion, what would you regard as the ideal number of children for the average Canadian family today?
    1 1 child
    2 2 children
    3 3 children
    4 4 children
    5 5 children
    6 6 or more children
    0 Non-response
    7 No opinion (Skip to Q. 21)
    8 No children (Skip to Q. 21)

20. (b) How many boys and girls would this be?
(FOR *PARTIAL* SEX PREFERENCE PUT SPECIFIC NUMBERS IN "BOYS" AND/OR "GIRLS" CATEGORY. PUT *UNSPECIFIED* REMAINDER IN "NO PREFERENCE" CATEGORY)
    Boys ____________ Number
    Girls ____________ Number
    No Preference ____________ Number
CHECK IF:
    Doesn't care ☐
    Not applicable ☐

21. (a) How about families with *one* less child than the number you consider ideal? Would ____ (1 LESS THAN THE IDEAL NUMBER IN Q. 20(a)) be too few?
    1 Yes (Skip to Q. 23)
    2 No
    3 Indifferent

21. (b) How about *two* less than your ideal?
    1 Yes
    2 No
    3 Indifferent

22. How many children would there have to be in a family before you would say there are *too many*?
    NUMBER ____________
    CHECK IF: No opinion; doesn't specify ☐

23. Have you and your husband ever talked about how many children each of you wants?
    1 Yes
    2 No
    0 Don't remember, won't say

24. (a) If you/your husband were to start married life over again how many children in all would you want to have?

Wife	0	1	2	3	4	5	6	7	8+	Don't know
Husband	0	1	2	3	4	5	6	7	8+	Don't know

IF "DON'T KNOW" SKIP TO Q. 25(a)

24. (b) What is the *main* reason that you would *not* want to have more than ________ children?
    1 Economic — general (cannot afford more, support more)
    2 Economic — education (cannot afford to educate more)
    3 Health of mother — physical or mental
    4 Practical — time for children (cannot give enough time if more)
    5 Practical — want more time for self and/or husband
    6 Other (Specify) ____________________
    0 Non-response

25. (a) Are you expecting now?
    1 Yes
    2 No
    3 Uncertain (PROBE FOR "YES" or "NO")

25. (b) IF "YES": How many months pregnant are you?
    Months ____________ (Skip to Q. 29)

26. (a) Do you have any reason to believe that you and your husband could not have another child if you wanted to?
    1 Yes
    2 No (Skip to Q. 28(a))
    3 Uncertain (Skip to Q. 28(a))

26. (b) IF "YES": What is your reason for believing you can't have another child?
    1 Told so by a doctor

2 Wife had operation to prevent pregnancy
3 Husband had operation to prevent pregnancy
4 Other (Specify) ____________

27. How long has it been since you have known, or been aware, that you could not have more children?
Months ________ and years ________
CHECK IF UNCERTAIN ☐

28. (a) Do you think you'll probably have a/another child? (IF "HOPE SO" OR "HOPE NOT" PROBE:) Well, do you think you're likely to have a/another child?
1 Yes
2 No (Skip to Q. 28(c))
3 Other (Specify) ____________

28. (b) How soon would you like to have your next child?
1 Within a year; as soon as possible (Skip to Q. 29)
2 1 year to 1 year 11 months from now
3 2 years to 2 years 11 months from now
4 Three years or more from now
5 No preference, don't care
6 Do not want more
7 Don't know

28. (c) Do you think you can avoid having a baby (before then)?
1 Yes
2 No
3 Uncertain

29. (a) Now, how many live-born children altogether have you had, including those that may have died?

0 1 2 3 4 5 6 7 8+

29. (b) IF "0": How many pregnancies have you had that did not result in a live birth?
NUMBER ____________ (Skip to Q. 38)
COMPLETE BIRTH RECORD (QUESTIONS 30–36) FOR ALL WOMEN WHO HAD ANY CHILDREN, i.e. CODED 1–8+ ABOVE.

Birth Record

ASK QUESTIONS 30–36 ONE BABY AT A TIME UNTIL *ALL* CHILDREN ARE ENTERED. (USE EXTRA SHEET IF NECESSARY)

		Code	1st	2nd	3rd	4th	5th	6th	7th	8th	9th	10th
30.	What did you name your (first) child?											
31.	Sex?	M (1) F (2)	1 2	1 2	1 2	1 2	1 2	1 2	1 2	1 2	1 2	1 2
32.	Date of Birth?	Day										
		Month										
		Year										
33.	Did you breast-feed (NAME)?	Yes 1 No 2	1 2	1 2	1 2	1 2	1 2	1 2	1 2	1 2	1 2	1 2
34.	IF "YES" For how many months?	Months										
35.	Is (NAME) still living?	Yes 1 No 2	1 2	1 2	1 2	1 2	1 2	1 2	1 2	1 2	1 2	1 2
36.	IF NOT LIVING When did (NAME) die?	Month Year										

37. (a) How many pregnancies have you had that did not result in a live birth?

0 1 2 3 4 5 6 7 8+

37. (b) IF MORE THAN "0" ASK: When, i.e. between the births of which children, did this (these) occur?

		Between								After
	Before 1st	1 & 2nd	2 & 3rd	3 & 4th	4 & 5th	5 & 6th	6 & 7th	7 & 8th	8th and last born	last born
Number of Pregnancies										

38. (a) If you could start life over again, at what age would you prefer to marry?

_______________ Age (PROBE FOR EXACT AGE)
_______________ Other Response (Specify) ________

38. (b) If you could go back to the time you were first married and start over again, how many children would you prefer to have by now?

_______________ (NUMBER)
CHECK IF NO PREFERENCE ☐
(IF PREFERENCE "0" OR "NO PREFERENCE" SKIP TO Q. 40)

39. What would be your preference according to sex?
ENTER NUMBERS: Boys ________ Girls ________
CHECK HERE IF NO PREFERENCE ☐

40. How long after marriage would you prefer/have preferred to wait for the first child?
Months ________ Years ________
CHECK HERE IF NO PREFERENCE ☐

41. In your opinion how many months or years should there ideally be between children? (IF DIFFERENT TIMES GIVEN, TAKE AVERAGE)
Months ________ Years ________
CHECK IF NO OPINION OR NON-RESPONSE ☐
(IF PREGNANT SKIP TO Q. 42(b))

42. (a) In addition to the children that you have now, how many more do you expect? CIRCLE ONE:

0 1 2 3 4 5 6 7 8+ Don't know.

42. (b) IF PREGNANT ASK: In addition to the child you are now expecting, how many more do you expect to have? CIRCLE ONE:

0 1 2 3 4 5 6 7 8+ Don't know.

43. Do you think that the number you actually will have might be greater than this or what? (PROBE IF NECESSARY)
   1 Definitely will be the same
   2 Probably will be the same
   3 Definitely will not exceed by *more* than 1
   4 Definitely will not exceed by *more* than 2
   5 Might exceed by more than two, cannot be sure
   Other (Specify) ____________

   IF NEVER PREGNANT SKIP TO Q. 46

44. (a) Did your last pregnancy occur because you *intentionally* tried to have a child at that time?
   1 Yes (Skip to Q. 46)
   2 No
   0 Non-response

44. (b) In what year did that pregnancy begin? ____________
   CHECK IF: Uncertain ☐ Non-response ☐

45. At that time, would you/your husband have preferred to have your pregnancy earlier, sometime later, or to have avoided it altogether?

Wife	*Husband*	
1	1	Preferred earlier
2	2	Preferred later
3	3	Preferred to avoid
4	4	Same time
5	5	Don't know, no opinion
0	0	Non-response

46. How many children — boys and girls — did your mother bear alive, including you?
   NUMBER OF: Boys ________ Girls ________
   CHECK IF DON'T KNOW ☐

47. How many brothers and sisters did you have at home most of the time when you were about 12 years of age?
   (Number) ________
   CHECK IF DON'T KNOW ☐

48. How many children did your husband's mother bear alive, including him?

NUMBER OF: Boys ________ Girls ________

CHECK IF DON'T KNOW ☐

49. How many brothers and sisters did your husband have in the house when he was about 12 years of age?

(Number) ________

CHECK IF DON'T KNOW ☐

50. Were you/was your husband the first born in the family, or what? (TREAT TWINS AS A SINGLE ORDER)

Wife	*Husband*	
9	9	Only child (Skip to Q. 52)
1	1	1st born
2	2	2nd born
3	3	3rd born
4	4	4th born
5	5	5th born
6	6	6th+ born
7	7	Don't know
0	0	Non-response

51. How much older or younger were you/your husband than your/his brothers and sisters nearest in age?

Next Older

Wife	*Husband*	*Difference in Age*
1	1	11 months or less
2	2	1 to 2 years 11 months
3	3	3 to 4 years 11 months
4	4	5 or more years
0	0	Not applicable, Don't know

Next Younger

Wife	*Husband*	*Difference in Age*
1	1	11 months or less
2	2	1 to 2 years 11 months
3	3	3 to 4 years 11 months
4	4	5 or more years
0	0	Not applicable, Don't know

52. How old were you/your husband when you first left school?

Wife	*Husband*	
1	1	14 or less

2	2	15–17
3	3	18–20
4	4	21 or older
5	5	Still attending
6	6	Don't know
0	0	Non-response

53. What was the highest grade or level of schooling that you/your husband ever attended? (ASK FOREIGN EDUCATED TO ESTIMATE ONTARIO EQUIVALENT)

Wife	*Husband*	
1	1	8th grade or less
2	2	9–10
3	3	11
4	4	12
5	5	13
6	6	Some university
7	7	Degree
		Other (Specify) ________________

54. Did you/your husband successfully complete that grade?

Wife	*Husband*	
1	1	No
2	2	Yes
0	0	Don't know, Won't say, Not applicable

55. In what province or country did you/your husband last attend school full time?

Wife ________________ *Husband* ________________

56. In what course, or field, were you/your husband when you last left school? (RECORD HIGHEST ATTAINED)

Wife	*Husband*	
1	1	*Elementary School* or less
		Secondary School
2	2	General Matriculation
3	3	Commercial–Technical
		Other (Specify) ________________
		Post Secondary: Non-University
5	5	Primary Teacher's College
6	6	Nursing School
		Other (Specify) ________________
		University
10	10	Law, Medicine

11	11	Science (including social)
12	12	Arts, Humanities
13	13	Secondary Teachers' College
		Other (Specify) ________

If you/your husband were educated in a foreign system to which the above does not apply, specify which system ________

____

57. (a) Did you/your husband take any courses of instruction in the past year, such as night school, correspondence, or any others?

Wife	*Husband*	
1	1	Yes
2	2	No

57. (b) IF "YES": What course(s) did you/your husband take? Where did you/he take it (them)?

	Wife	*Husband*
Name of Course(s)	________	________
Institution(s)		
Where taken	________	________

58. Are you/your husband taking any such courses this year?

Wife	*Husband*	
1	1	Yes
2	2	No

59. Would you/your husband call yourself Protestant, Roman Catholic, Jewish, or what?

Wife	*Husband*	
1	1	Protestant
2	2	Roman Catholic (Skip to Q. 61)
3	3	Jewish (Skip to Q. 61)
		Other (Specify) ________

60. What denomination are you?

Wife	*Husband*	
1	1	Anglican
2	2	United Church
3	3	Presbyterian
4	4	Methodist
5	5	Baptist
6	6	Lutheran
7	7	Greek Orthodox
8	8	Ukrainian Catholic
		Other (Specify) ________

61. Did you/your husband ever belong to another religion or denomination?

Wife	*Husband*	
1	1	Yes
2	2	No (Skip to Q. 64)
0	0	Non-response

62. When did you/your husband change your religion or denomination? Was it (READ CATEGORIES)

Wife	*Husband*	
1	1	Before you met?
2	2	Since you met but before marriage?
3	3	Since marriage?
0	0	Don't know, won't say

63. What kind of change was it?

0 Respondent won't say, doesn't know

Husband only changed

1 From R.C. to Protestant
2 From Protestant to R.C.
3 Other

Wife only changed

4 From R.C. to Protestant
5 From Protestant to R.C.
6 Other

Both changed

7 From R.C. to Protestant
8 From Protestant to R.C.
9 Other

64. How often in an average fall or winter *month* do you/does your husband attend religious services?

Wife	*Husband*	
1	1	Don't attend
2	2	Once or twice or less
3	3	Three or four times
4	4	Five or more times
0	0	Non-response

65. About how far away is your church?

Wife	*Husband*	
1	1	Less than 1 mile
2	2	1–3 miles
3	3	More than 3 miles
		Other (Specify) ______________

66. Did you/your husband mostly attend a Separate primary school (i.e. R.C.), a public supported school, or what?

Wife	*Husband*	
1	1	Separate (R.C.)
2	2	Other Private
3	3	Public (Gov't)
		Other (Specify) ________________

67. Was there any Separate (R.C.) primary school in your/your husband's community at that time?

Wife	*Husband*	
1	1	Yes
2	2	No
0	0	Don't know

68. (ASK OF *BOTH* IF EITHER/BOTH *NOW* R.C.: IF NEITHER *NOW* R.C. SKIP TO Q. 72) Assuming one to be available, do you/does your husband feel that your children should go to a Separate primary school?

Wife	*Husband*	
1	1	Yes
2	2	No
0	0	No opinion, Don't know

69. Why do you/does your husband feel this way? (CIRCLE ONLY *MAIN* REASON)

Wife	*Husband*	
		Reason for:
1	1	Want religious education
2	2	Better discipline
3	3	Better instruction
4	4	Advised to by priest
		Other (Specify) ________________
		Reason against:
6	6	Type of discipline
7	7	Poor instruction
		Other (Specify) ________________

70. (TO BE ASKED IF RESPONDENT HAS OR HAS HAD CHILDREN OF SCHOOL AGE – SEE Q. 32 – OTHERWISE SKIP TO Q. 72) Have any of your children *ever* attended or are any *now* attending a Separate school?

1 Yes
2 No

71. Is there a Separate school nearby or easily accessible?
    1 Yes
    2 No
    0 Don't know

72. Was your husband at work last week?
    1 Yes (Skip to Q. 74)
    2 No
    0 Don't know, Won't say

73. IF NOT AT WORK LAST WEEK: What was the reason?
    1 Temporarily absent due to illness
    2 Temporarily absent on leave or vacation
    3 Disabled
    4 Retired
    5 Unemployed
    6 Student
    7 On Strike
    0 Other (Specify) ________________

74. Does he operate his own business, that is work for himself, or does he work in a business, government agency, or for someone else?
    1 Self employed (Skip to Q. 76)
    2 Employee
    0 Don't know, Won't say

75. For whom does he work (or last worked if not now working)?

    ____

    Name of firm, company, agency etc.

    ____

    Department, division, branch, section

76. What kind of business or industry is this?

    ____

77. What kind of work does he do in his job? (PROBE FULLY)

____

____

78. Is this his usual occupation?
    1 Yes (Skip to Q. 80)
    2 No
    0 Don't know, won't say

79. IF "NO": What is his usual job? DESCRIBE FULLY: IF NO USUAL OCCUPATION CHECK: ☐

____

____

80. (a) Approximately what is his annual income before taxes and other deductions from all sources, such as wages and salary, commissions, bonuses, interests, dividends, etc.? (SHOW CARD A)

1 Less than $1500
2 1500–2999
3 3000–3999
4 4000–4999
5 5000–5999
6 6000–7999
7 8000–9999
8 10,000–11,999
9 12,000–14,999
10 15,000 and above
11 Don't know (Skip to Q. 81)
00 Non-response, Refused (Skip to Q. 81)

80. (b) (INTERVIEWER: EVALUATE IMPRESSION OF INCOME RESPONSE BY CIRCLING ONE OF THE FOLLOWING)

1 Appears very certain
2 Appears somewhat certain
3 Appears somewhat uncertain
4 Appears very uncertain

81. About how many weeks or months was your husband out of work during the past year?

1 None
2 Less than a week
3 A week to less than 2 months
4 2 to 3 months
5 More than 3 months
6 Don't know
0 Won't say

82. At the time you were married was your husband working at a full time job, or what?

1 Full time job

2 Student (Skip to Q. 84)
3 Non student, unemployed or part time job
0 Don't know, won't say

83. Did he operate his own business or work for someone else?
1 Self-employed
2 Employee
0 Don't know, won't say

84. For whom did your husband work at the time you were first married or in his first job after marriage?

____

Firm, agency etc.

____

Department, Division etc.

85. What kind of business or industry was that?

____

86. What kind of work did he do? (PROBE FULLY)

____

____

87. (a) Approximately what was his annual income at that time before tax and other deductions from all sources, such as wages, salary, commissions, bonuses, interests, dividends etc.? (SHOW CARD A)
1 Less than $1500
2 1500–2999
3 3000–3999
4 4000–4999
5 5000–5999
6 6000–7999
7 8000–9999
8 10,000–11,999
9 12,000–14,999
10 15,000 and above
11 Don't know
00 Non-response, Refused

87. (b) (INTERVIEWER: EVALUATE IMPRESSION OF INCOME RESPONSE BY CIRCLING ONE OF THE FOLLOWING)
1 Appears very certain

2	Appears somewhat certain
3	Appears somewhat uncertain
4	Appears very uncertain

88. At the time of your marriage, was your/your husband's father self-employed, or did he work for someone else?

Wife's Father	*Husband's Father*	
1	1	Self-employed (Skip to Q. 90)
2	2	Employee
3	3	Unemployed
4	4	Retired, deceased
0	0	Don't know; won't say

89. For whom did your/your husband's father work at the time of your marriage (or for whom did he work last)?

Wife's Father	*Husband's Father*
____________________	____________________
Firm, Agency etc.	Firm, Agency etc.
____________________	____________________
Department, Division etc.	Department, Division etc.

90. What kind of business or industry was that?

Wife's Father	*Husband's Father*
____________________	____________________

91. What kind of work did he do?

Wife's Father	*Husband's Father*
____________________	____________________
____________________	____________________

92. What was the highest level of education completed by your/your husband's father?

Wife's Father	*Husband's Father*	
1	1	Elementary only
2	2	Some high school or secondary
3	3	High school graduate
4	4	Some university
5	5	University graduate
6	6	Other post secondary
7	7	*No equivalent; foreign system*
0	0	Don't know; won't say

93. Did you have a job before you were married?
   1 Yes
   2 No (Skip to Q. 100)
   0 Don't remember, won't say

94. For whom did you work?

   ____
   Firm, agency, etc.

   ____
   Department, division, etc.

95. What kind of business or industry was this?

   ____

96. What kind of work did you do?

   ____
   ____

97. Was that job full time — that is 7 or more hours per day and 5 or more days per week — or what? (READ CATEGORIES IF NECESSARY)
   1 Full time (AS DESCRIBED ABOVE)
   2 Regular part time, 7 or more hours/day, less than 5 days a week
   3 Occasional part time, less than 7 hours/day, less than 5 days/week
   4 All other work arrangements
   0 Don't remember, won't say

98. Approximately how much did you earn per week (or per month) before any deductions at that time? (USE CARD B)

	Per Week		*Per Month*
1	Less than $25	1	Less than $100
2	25–39	2	100–159
3	40–59	3	160–239
4	60–79	4	240–319
5	80–99	5	320–399
6	100–124	6	400–499
7	125–149	7	500–599
8	150–199	8	600–799
9	200–249	9	800–999
10	250+	10	1000+

11	Don't know	11	Don't know
00	Non-response	00	Non-response

99. (a) For how long after marriage did you *continue* to work before stopping to have children or for some other reason?
    Months ________ Years ________

99. (b) IF DID NOT STOP, WORKED CONTINUOUSLY SINCE MARRIAGE
    CHECK HERE ☐

100. Were you attending school full time at the time of your marriage?
    1 Yes
    2 No

101. Are you working now at a job outside your home?
    1 Yes (Skip to Q. 104)
    2 No

102. Are you actively looking for a job?
    1 Yes
    2 No (Skip to Q. 109)

103. IF LOOKING FOR A JOB, What steps have you actually taken? (CIRCLE ALL APPLICABLE)
    1 Registered with N.E.S.
    2 Contacts with employers
    3 Placed ad. in newspaper
    Other activity (Specify) ____________________
    Skip to Q. 109

104. For whom are you working?

    ____
    Firm, agency, etc.

    ____
    Department, division, etc.

105. What kind of business or industry is this?

    ____

106. What kind of work do you do?

    ____
    ____

107. Is this a full-time job — i.e. 7 or more hours per day and 5 or more days per week, or what? (READ CATEGORIES IF NECESSARY)

1 Full time: AS NOTED ABOVE
2 Regular part-time: 7 or more hours/day less than 5 days/week
3 Occasional part-time: Less than 7 hours/ less than 5 days/week
4 All other work arrangements
0 Doesn't remember, won't say

108. What is your approximate income before deductions? (SHOW CARD B)

Per Week
1 Less than $25
2 25–39
3 40–59
4 60–79
5 80–99
6 100–124
7 125–149
8 150–199
9 200–249
10 250+
11 Doesn't remember
00 Won't say

Per Month
1 Less than $100
2 100–159
3 160–239
4 240–319
5 320–399
6 400–499
7 500–599
8 600–799
9 800–999
10 1,000+
11 Doesn't remember
00 Won't say

We would like to fill in your work history since marriage.
Let's start at the beginning. (ASK "2nd last to last child" INTERVAL *ONLY* IF *MORE THAN* 4 CHILDREN. IF INTERVAL NOT APPLICABLE, LEAVE Q. 109 AND 110 *BLANK*; DO *NOT* CHECK "NO WORK" OR "N.A.")

	Question	*Marriage to First Child (OR UNTIL NOW IF NO LIVE BIRTHS)*	*First Child to 2nd Child*	*2nd Child to 3rd Child*	*3rd Child to 4th Child*	*2nd Last to Last Child*	*Last Child to Now*
109.	How long did you work altogether from:?	Months—— Years —— IF NO WORK CHECK ☐	Months—— Years —— IF NO WORK CHECK ☐	Months—— Years —— IF NO WORK CHECK ☐	Months—— Years —— IF NO WORK CHECK ☐	Months—— Years —— IF NO WORK CHECK ☐	Months—— Years —— IF NO WORK CHECK ☐
110.	How regularly did you work? ENTER MOST REGULAR EMPLOYMENT	Full time........1 Reg. pt. time..2 Occ. pt. time..3 Other.............4 Non-response, N.A................0	1 2 3 4 0	1 2 3 4 0	1 2 3 4 0	1 2 3 4 0	1 2 3 4 0

(SEE Q. 107 FOR WORK CATEGORIES)

111. Do you own or rent your present home?
  1 Rent
  2 Own
  3 Other arrangement

112. On an average week or month, approximately how much do you set aside or spend from the family's take home income, for: (CHECK ALL THAT APPLY)

	$	Week	Month	Non-Resp.	Don't Know	EVALUATE CERTAINTY OF RESPONSE: Very Unsure	EVALUATE CERTAINTY OF RESPONSE: Reasonably Sure
Rent or mortgage	—.00	☐	☐	☐	☐	☐	☐
All other time payments	—.00	☐	☐	☐	☐	☐	☐
Car payments alone	—.00	☐	☐	☐	☐	☐	☐
Food & other consumables	—.00	☐	☐	☐	☐	☐	☐
Savings	—.00	☐	☐	☐	☐	☐	☐

113. How many cars do you and your husband own?
  0 None (Skip to Q. 115)
  1 One
  2 Two
  3 Three or more

114. (a) Do you have seat belts in your car? (NEWEST CAR)
  1 Yes
  2 No (Skip to Q. 115)
  3 Don't know (Skip to Q. 115)

114. (b) How often do you wear them?
  1 All the time
  2 Most of the time
  3 Sometimes
  4 Infrequently
  5 Never

115. Whatever it is you feel you want out of life, how closely do you feel that you are approaching it?
  1 Very closely
  2 Fairly closely
  3 Only to some extent
  4 Not at all
  0 Non-response

116. In general what kind of success do you feel you and your husband are having financially? (READ CATEGORIES)
 1 Very good
 2 Good
 3 Fair
 4 Poor
 0 Non-response

117. Some people make very definite plans about the future, planning their lives in many respects for several years ahead, while others do not. How about you? Do you: (READ CATEGORIES)
 1 Generally plan most things
 2 Plan some things — leave others to chance
 3 Seldom plan ahead
 4 Take things as they come; don't plan
 0 Non-response

118. Suppose your husband lost his job tomorrow and neither he nor you could find work for one month. Do you feel that you could manage to pay all your usual bills for that month out of the family savings?
 1 Yes
 2 No
 3 Unsure
 0 Non-response

119. How often do you deny yourself and your family things you and they would like because of provisions you are making for the future? (READ CATEGORIES)
 1 Often
 2 Sometimes
 3 Seldom or never
 0 Non-response

120. How about your husband, how often does he do this? Would you say: (READ CATEGORIES)
 1 Often
 2 Sometimes
 3 Seldom or never
 0 Non-response

121. What year is your car? (RECORD *NEWEST* IF MORE THAN ONE)
 Year ________
 7 Don't know
 8 No car (Skip to Q. 123)
 0 Non-response

122. When do you/does he plan to replace that car?
 Year ________
 7 Don't know
 0 Non-response, Not applicable

123. Do you expect any of your children to continue schooling after high school?
 1 Yes
 2 No (Skip to Q. 125)
 3 Uncertain
 4 Not applicable (Skip to Q. 125)
 0 Non-response (Skip to Q. 125)

124. Have you taken any steps yet to finance this education? (IF "NO" CIRCLE "NONE"; IF "YES" ASK "What steps?"
 1 None
 2 Savings: Baby Bonus
 3 Savings: Other sources
 4 Insurance Plan
 5 Savings plus insurance
 6 Other (Specify) ____________________
 0 Non-response

125. How often do you or your husband personally put aside money for savings or investment *beyond* anything provided by your employer, such as pension plans, health and insurance, annuities etc.?
 1 Regularly, such as every month
 2 Often, but not on a regular basis
 3 Occasionally, no regular plan
 4 Seldom or never
 0 Non-response

126. Many couples use contraceptives to limit the size of their family or to have their children when they want them. We would like to hear some of your views on this subject.

First, in general, do you approve of married couples doing something to plan their families? (PROBE)

1 Yes
2 All right for others (up to individual)
3 No
0 Non-response

127. How does your husband feel about it?

1 Approve
2 Disapprove
3 Husband ambivalent
4 Wife not sure what he thinks
0 Non-response

128. IF WIFE "NO" OR HUSBAND "DISAPPROVES" OR "AMBIVALENT" ASK: Do you/does your husband approve of the rhythm method?

Wife	*Husband*	
1	1	Yes
2	2	No
3	3	Don't know
0	0	Non-response

129. (a) Assuming a woman's average menstrual cycle is 28 days, on what day, if any, counting from the *beginning* of her period, is she most likely to become pregnant? (IF RANGE GIVEN USE BRACKETS BUT PROBE FULLY FOR SPECIFIC DAY)

1 2 3 4 5 6 7 8 9 10 11 12
13 14 15 16 17 18 19 20 21 22 23 24
25 26 27 28 Don't know

129. (b) Have you ever made a temperature chart in order to find out on which days you are more likely to become pregnant? (CIRCLE ONE)

1 Yes
2 No

Here is a card listing by number some of the commonly used methods of birth control. (SHOW CARD TO RESPONDENT)

	Q. 130	*Q. 131 (FOR "THOSE KNOWN") ASK:*				*Q. 132*	*Q. 133*
	Which of these do you know about? (CHECK THOSE KNOWN)	*How effective are these in preventing pregnancies? (READ METHODS KNOWN)*				*Are you* now *using any of these for contraception? (CHECK ALL* NOW *USED)*	*Have you ever used any other for contraception? (CHECK ALL OTHERS EVER USED)*
Method		*Very Effective*	*Somewhat Effective*	*Not Effective*	*Don't Know*		
1. Rhythm (safe period)							
2. Withdrawal (pulling out)							
3. Oral Pills							
4. Diaphragm							
5. Jelly, Cream, Foam							
6. Suppositories							
7. Condom (rubber or safe)							
8. I.U.D. (loop, coil)							
9. Douching							
10. Abstinence							
11. Other (SPECIFY)							

134. (IF *NEVER* USED ANY METHOD SKIP TO Q. 161)
IF *NOW* USING OR *EVER* USED ANY METHOD ASK:
How old were you when you first used any of the above methods?

Age ________
1 Don't remember
0 Non-response

(IF NEVER USED THE PILL ASK: Have you ever used the pill for medical purposes? IF STILL "NO" SKIP TO Q. 157)

135. How did you first come to know about the pill?
(IF UNABLE TO SINGLE OUT ONE SOURCE, CIRCLE "DON'T REMEMBER")

1 Husband
2 Friend or relative
3 Doctor
4 Nurse
5 Social worker
6 Magazine, newspaper or other printed materials
7 T.V., radio
8 Other means or person
9 Don't remember
0 Non-response

136. (a) Have you used the pill chiefly to prevent pregnancy or for some other reason?

1 To prevent pregnancy
2 For menstrual disorders
3 For both these reasons
Other reason (Specify) ____________________
0 Non-response

136. (b) (IF NO CHILDREN, SKIP TO Q. 137) Did you use the pill before the birth of your last child?

1 Yes
2 No
3 Uncertain
0 Non-response

137. Here is a calendar (GIVE CALENDAR TO RESPONDENT). To the best of your knowledge, during what months and years have you used the pill?

	Winter		*Spring*			*Summer*			*Fall*			
Year	*Jan*	*Feb*	*Mar*	*Apr*	*May*	*Jun*	*Jul*	*Aug*	*Sep*	*Oct*	*Nov*	*Dec*
1959	1	2	3	4	5	6	7	8	9	10	11	12
1960	1	2	3	4	5	6	7	8	9	10	11	12
1961	1	2	3	4	5	6	7	8	9	10	11	12
1962	1	2	3	4	5	6	7	8	9	10	11	12
1963	1	2	3	4	5	6	7	8	9	10	11	12
1964	1	2	3	4	5	6	7	8	9	10	11	12
1965	1	2	3	4	5	6	7	8	9	10	11	12
1966	1	2	3	4	5	6	7	8	9	10	11	12
1967	1	2	3	4	5	6	7	8	9	10	11	12
1968	1	2	3	4	5	6	7	8	9	10	11	12

138. How certain are you about the year and the month when you *first* used the pill?

Year	*Month*	
1	1	Very certain
2	2	Fairly certain
3	3	Uncertain

139. What is the *main* reason you *first* tried the pill?
   1 To regulate menstrual disorder
   2 Most effective method
   3 Most convenient to use
   4 Other (Specify) ______________________
   0 Non-response

140. About how old was the doctor who gave you your first prescription for the pill, that is, how old was the doctor *at that time*? (IF VAGUE READ AGE GROUPS)
   1 Under 35
   2 35–39
   3 40–49
   4 50–59
   5 60 plus
   6 Don't remember
   0 Non-response

141. Do you know the brand name of the pill you are *now* taking or *last* used?

(IF RESPONDENT CANNOT REMEMBER SHOW THE LIST TO HER)

1 Enovid
2 Enovid-E
3 Ovulen
4 Norinyl
5 Norlestrin
6 Ortho-Novum
7 Provest or Secrovin
8 C-Quens
9 Oracon
10 Lyndiol
11 Ovral
12 None of above
13 Don't know
00 Non-response

142. Have you ever used any other brands? If so, which ones?

Brands: 1 2 3 4 5 6 7 8 9 10 11 12 13 00

CHECK IF NEVER USED OTHER BRAND ☐

143. Since you first began using the pill have you ever stopped use intentionally?

1 Yes
2 No (Skip to Q. 147)
0 Non-response

144. When you last stopped intentionally, what were your reasons? (CIRCLE *ALL* THAT APPLY)

1 Wanted to become pregnant (Skip to Q. 147)
2 Wanted to lose weight
3 Didn't feel well when taking: headaches, nausea
4 Spotting
5 Depression
6 Worried over threat to health
7 Too expensive
8 Couldn't remember to take pill
9 Other (Specify) ______________________
0 Non-response

145. When you stopped, did you continue with some form of contraception?

1 Yes
2 No (Skip to Q. 147)
3 Don't remember
0 Non-response

146. What method(s) did you substitute? (CIRCLE ALL THAT APPLY)
1 Rhythm (safe period)
2 Withdrawal
3 Oral pills
4 Diaphragm
5 Jelly, cream, foam
6 Suppositories
7 Condom (rubber
8 I.U.D. (loop, coil)
9 Douching
10 Abstinence
11 Other (Specify) ____________________
00 Non-response

147. Did you ever run out of pills because you forgot to renew your prescription or because you didn't get to the drugstore in time?
1 Yes
2 No (Skip to Q. 150)
3 Don't remember
0 Non-response

148. Did you then use some other method?
1 Yes
2 No
3 Don't remember
0 Non-response

149. Did you become pregnant on this occasion?
1 Yes
2 No

ASK ONLY OF WOMEN *NOW* USING THE PILL

150. How often in an average month do you forget to take your pill at the proper time and remember only after *24 hrs. or more*? (IF "LESS THAN ONCE A MONTH" ASK "IN AN AVERAGE YEAR")
1 Twice a year or less

2 3–6 times a year
3 7–11 times a year
4 Once a month
5 Twice a month
6 3 times a month
7 4 times a month or more
8 Never forget
9 Don't know
0 Non-response

151. (IF "NEVER FORGETS" SKIP TO Q. 152)
Did you use an additional method or abstain, for the remainder of the cycle in which you last missed taking a pill?
1 Yes
2 No
0 Non-response

152. For how many months was your last prescription for the pill? (CIRCLE *ONE*)
1 One month
2 Two–three
3 Four–five
4 Six
5 Seven–eleven
6 Twelve (one year)
7 More than one year
8 Can't remember, Don't know
0 Non-response

153. When you first began taking the pill, did the doctor examine your breasts or give you an internal examination?
1 Yes
2 No
0 Don't know, Non-response

154. (a) Does your doctor require an internal examination each time you have your prescription renewed?
1 Yes
2 No
3 Not applicable
0 Non-response, Don't know

154. (b) Did you have an internal examination the last time you had your prescription renewed?

1 Yes
2 No (Skip to Q. 155)
3 Not applicable (Skip to Q. 155)
0 Non-response, Don't know (Skip to Q. 155)

154. (c) Did this examination include a "Pap Smear" (Cancer smear)?
1 Yes
2 No
3 Don't know
0 Non-response

155. (a) Before taking the pill, what method if any, did you last use? (CIRCLE *ONE ONLY*)
1 Rhythm (safe period)
2 Withdrawal
3 Oral pills
4 Diaphragm
5 Jelly, cream, foam
6 Suppositories
7 Condom (Rubber)
8 I.U.D. (Loop, Coil)
9 Douching
10 Abstinence
11 Other (Specify) ______
00 Non-response
CHECK IF NO METHOD ☐
ASK (b) AND SKIP TO Q. 157

155. (b) Did you not use any method because you:
(READ CATEGORIES)
1 Were not married then
2 Wanted to become pregnant
3 Were unconcerned about pregnancy
4 Other
0 Non-response

156. (a) Before that what methods did you use?
1 Rhythm (safe period)
2 Withdrawal
3 Oral pills
4 Diaphragm
5 Jelly, cream, foam
6 Suppositories

7 Condom (Rubber)
8 I.U.D. (Loop, Coil)
9 Douching
10 Abstinence
11 Other (Specify) ______________________
00 Non-response
CHECK IF NO METHOD ☐

156. (b) Did you not use any method because you: (READ CATEGORIES)
1 Were not married then
2 Wanted to become pregnant
3 Were unconcerned about pregnancy
4 Other
0 Non-response

157. How many times have you become pregnant while using contraception?
0 Never (Skip to Q. 161)
1 1
2 2
3 3
4 4
5 5
6 6+
7 Not sure
0 Non-response

158. When did this (these) pregnancies *begin*, that is, in what year?
Year(s) __________
____
____
____

159. On the *last* occasion when you became pregnant while using contraception, what method were you using?
2 Rhythm (safe period)
3 Withdrawal
4 Oral pills
5 Diaphragm
6 Jelly, cream, foam
7 Suppositories
8 Condom (Rubber)

9 I.U.D. (Loop, Coil)
10 Douching
11 Abstinence
12 Other (Specify) ______________
00 Non-response

160. Do you think you may have become pregnant then because you took a chance sometime?
1 Yes
2 No

161. (IF *EVER* USED THE PILL, SKIP TO Q. 162. *IF NEVER USED*, ASK:) What is the *main* reason you never tried the pill? (CIRCLE ONLY *MAIN* REASON)
1 Wife or husband does not approve of any contraception
2 Doesn't care about protection
3 Wants to become pregnant
4 Satisfied with other methods
5 Believe pill ineffective
6 Believe pill a health hazard
7 Object to side effects
8 Too expensive
9 Might forget to take
10 Husband has objection to pill
11 Religious objections
12 Other (Specify) ______________
00 Non-response

162. In the future, if you wanted to avoid pregnancy would you use the pill?
1 Yes (Skip to Q. 164)
2 No
3 Uncertain

163. (a) Why do you think you would *not* use the pill in the future?
1 Religious objections to contraception
2 Sterile or subfecund, too old to conceive
3 Objectionable side effects
4 Health hazard
5 Difficult to take as directed
6 Too expensive
7 Satisfied with present methods
Other (Specify) ______________

163. (b) How much does a month's supply of pills cost?
$__.00
CHECK HERE IF "DON'T KNOW" ☐

164. Many people think that if a couple already has more children than they can feed, clothe and house, and then the wife gets pregnant again, the couple should be allowed to have an abortion performed by a doctor. Other people think it is wrong for a pregnant woman to have an abortion under any circumstances. We would like to have your views on this issue.
Suppose the couple could afford another child but felt strongly that they did not want another one; would you approve of their having an abortion if the wife accidentally became pregnant?
1 Yes
2 No
3 Don't know

165. Suppose the couple is very poor and having another child would mean extreme economic hardships. If the wife became accidentally pregnant would you approve of their having an abortion?
1 Yes
2 No
3 Don't know

166. Here are some situations in which some people think it is all right for the woman to have an abortion if it is performed under proper medical conditions. Under which of these would you say an abortion is all right. SHOW CARD TO RESPONDENT (CHECK ALL THAT APPLY). THEN ASK part h.

	Agree	*Disagree*	*Unsure*
a. Having a child would endanger the mother's life	☐	☐	☐
b. There is a strong chance of a deformed or mentally handicapped child	☐	☐	☐
c. Pregnancy due to rape	☐	☐	☐
d. Unmarried and does not wish to marry the father, or father refuses to marry	☐	☐	☐

e. Serious marriage difficulties likely to result in divorce	☐	☐	☐
f. Mother mentally ill or retarded	☐	☐	☐
g. Mother would experience severe psychiatric and emotional problems if not aborted	☐	☐	☐
h. Are there any others? (Specify) ______	☐	☐	☐

167. If you should accidentally become pregnant and already had all the children you want, do you think you might consider having an abortion to terminate the pregnancy if abortion for this reason were made legal in Canada?
 1 Yes
 2 No
 3 Uncertain

168. In your opinion should contraceptives be made readily available to unmarried persons: (READ 1 and 2)

	Yes	*No*	*Un-certain*	*No Response*
1. Who are aged 21 or more?	1	2	3	0
2. Who are under 21?	1	2	3	0

169. (a) In your opinion, is it all right for a man to have some experience of premarital sexual intercourse if: he *is engaged* to the woman? He *is not engaged* to the woman?

Engaged	*Not Engaged*	
1	1	Yes
2	2	Qualified "yes"
3	3	Qualified "no"
4	4	No
5	5	Don't know
0	0	No response

169. (b) In your opinion, is it all right for a woman to have some experience of premarital sexual intercourse if: she *is engaged* to the man? She *is not engaged* to the man?

Engaged	*Not Engaged*	
1	1	Yes
2	2	Qualified "yes"
3	3	Qualified "no"

4 4 No
5 5 Don't know
0 0 No response

ASK IF MORE THAN "0" in Q. 42(a) or (b)

170. (a) When do you plan to have your next/a child; that is, in how many months or years from now?

_____________ MONTHS _____________ YEARS

CHECK IF: DON'T KNOW; NO PLANS ☐
NO RESPONSE ☐

170. (b) By what age do you plan to have stopped having children?

_____________ AGE

CHECK IF: DON'T KNOW ☐
NO RESPONSE ☐

Appendix B

Multiple Classification Analysis of Family Size

As many of the socio-economic variables are interrelated, it is difficult to assess their relative importance as determinants of fertility performance without appropriate multivariate analysis. Because our data are at various levels of measurement, we have used a multivariate analysis technique called "Multiple Classification Analysis."[1] Basically this is an extension of multiple regression analysis to situations where the independent variables can be either in subclasses or discontinuous variables such as religion or nativity. In multiple classification analysis each subclass of an independent variable is a predictor. An advantage of multiple classification analysis is that no assumptions about linearity of the subclasses are required. The technique presents a mean value of the dependent variable for each subclass of each independent variable expressed as a deviation from the grand mean. Thus if the subclasses of a predictor variable make no difference in, say, number of children, then deviations from the mean number of children will all be zero for that predictor. If the predictor makes a difference, the deviations indicate how much of a difference. To illustrate: the grand mean for the current number of children is 2.26 (table 5); from table 23 we see that women age 18–24 have 1.11 fewer children than the average (or 2.26 − 1.11 = 1.15)

[1] Andrews, Morgan, and Sonquist, *Multiple Classification Analysis.*

and women 40 and over have more than the average number(2.26 + .38 = 2.64). Adjusted deviations which indicate what difference the predictor variable makes after taking account of other variables are interpreted in a similar fashion.

The Multiple Classification Analysis for current fertility is presented in table 68. Age and marriage duration are the two most powerful predictors. Adjusting for marriage duration reduces the variability by age, but the converse is not true. Marriage duration explains by and large most of the variation in current fertility.[2] As age and especially marriage duration have a predominant effect on current fertility, examination of other differentials should control for these variables. Such controls serve either to diminish or enhance a relationship depending on the correlation between a given predictor variable on the one hand and age, marital duration, and other variables on the other.

Differences by nativity status become more pronounced when the influence of age, marriage duration, and other factors is removed. In most other instances the relationships previously noted persist but are diminished. This is the case with respect to education, wife's religion and religiosity, and husband's occupation. The most important variable seems to be the wife's labour force status. Women in the labour force have considerably lower fertility than non-working women even after taking account of education, religion, husband's income, and nativity. However, it is difficult to establish a cause and effect relationship between fertility and labour force status.

For total expected family size (table 69), the basic pattern of relationships is essentially the same as for current fertility. Marriage duration does not have the same dominating influence on total expected fertility as on current fertility. However, it continues to be an important predictor. Women in the labour force expected to complete their family at a smaller size than women not in the labour force, even when all other factors including age and marriage duration are taken into account.

[2] To illustrate how tables 23 and 24 are to be read, for marriage duration, those women in the duration category 0–2 years will have 1.66 children less than the grand mean of 2.25 and 1.60 children less than the grand mean even if all the influences of other factors are removed. Because MCA ignores cases where no responses are available on any of the variables, small differences between the unadjusted deviations reported here with means presented earlier are possible. However, the overall trends and differentials revealed in the MCA analysis should be valid.

Table 68 Multiple Classification Analysis of Current Number of Children in Relation to Selected Demographic and Socio-Economic Characteristics

Predictors	*Unadjusted Deviations from Grand Mean*	*Deviations Adjusted for Age and Marriage Duration*	*Deviations Adjusted for All Other Predictors*	*Number of Women*
Age of Wife				
18–24	−1.11	.18 (a)	.11	197
25–29	− .59	.03 (a)	.00	322
30–34	.21	.16 (a)	.16	329
35–39	.49	.12 (a)	.13	358
40 and over	.38	− .32 (a)	− .28	426
Marriage Duration				
0–2 years	−1.66	−1.78 (b)	−1.60	156
3–5 years	− .94	−1.03 (b)	− .97	192
6–10 years	− .93	− .16 (b)	− .20	400
11–15 years	.47	.39 (b)	.34	380
16–20 years	.55	.68 (b)	.64	318
More than 20	.66	.95 (b)	.98	186
Nativity				
Native born	.02	.04	.08	957
Foreign born	− .03	− .06	− .12	674
Education of Wife				
Less than 8 years	.41	.26	.16	362
High school 1–3	.07	.04	.05	603
High school 4–5	− .25	− .19	− .15	476
College	− .37	− .12	− .07	190
Religion of Wife				
Protestant	− .10	− .10	− .08	974
Catholic	.25	.26	.21	498
Jewish	− .06	− .22	− .28	62
Others	− .20	− .08	− .04	96

Table 68 (Continued)

Predictors	*Unadjusted Deviations from Grand Mean*	*Deviations Adjusted for Age and Marriage Duration*	*Deviations Adjusted for All Other Predictors*	*Number of Women*
Wife's (Monthly) Church Attendance				
Don't attend	− .14	− .10	− .03	553
Once or twice or less	− .09	− .06	− .05	486
3–4 times	.17	.08	.02	397
5 or more	.27	.27	.17	196
Husband's Income				
Less than $4000	− .23	.00	− .02	112
$4000–$5999	.01	.12	.11	417
$6000–$7999	− .14	− .08	− .04	395
$8000–$9999	− .10	− .15	− .14	228
$10000–$11999	.03	− .13	− .12	180
$12000 or more	.36	.11	.10	182
D.K. and N.R.	.27	.17	.04	118
Husband's Occupation				
Upper white collar	.01	− .05	.00	616
Lower white collar	− .25	− .18	− .12	284
Blue collar	.09	.11	.05	732
Wife's Labour Force Status				
Working	− .45	− .38	− .37	585
Not working	.25	.21	.21	1046

(*a*) *Adjusted for marriage duration only.*
(*b*) *Adjusted for age only.*

Table 69 Multiple Classification Analysis of Total Expected Number of Children in Relation to Selected Demographic and Socio-Economic Characteristics

Predictors	*Unadjusted Deviations from Grand Mean*	*Deviations Adjusted for Age and Marriage Duration*	*Deviations Adjusted for All Other Predictors*	*Number of Women*
Age of Wife				
18–24	− .01	.46	.47	197
25–29	− .08	.27	.26	322
30–34	.06	.15 (a)	.15	329
35–39	.12	− .02	− .02	358
40 and over	− .08	− .52	− .52	426
Marriage Duration				
0–2 years	− .12	− .48	− .47	156
3–5 years	− .20	− .51	− .50	192
6–10 years	− .11	− .28 (b)	− .32	400
11–15 years	.08	.08	.08	380
16–20 years	.10	.40	.38	318
	.19	.67	.77	186
Nativity				
Native born	.05	.04	.09	957
Foreign born	− .07	− .06	− .12	674
Education of Wife				
Less than 8 years	.18	.14	.01	362
High school 1–3	.00	− .04	.00	603
High school 4–5	− .15	− .12	− .10	476
College	.07	.16	.22	190
Religion of Wife				
Protestant	− .13	− .13	− .12	974
Catholic	.29	.30	.26	498
Jewish	.01	− .01	− .03	62
Others	− .19	− .17	− .14	96

Table 69 (Continued)

Predictors	*Unadjusted Deviations from Grand Mean*	*Deviations Adjusted for Age and Marriage Duration*	*Deviations Adjusted for All Other Predictors*	*Number of Women*
Wife's (Monthly) Church Attendance				
Don't attend	− .17	− .18	− .10	553
Once or twice or less	− .05	− .05	− .03	486
3–4 times	.14	.14	.05	397
5 or more times	.30	.33	.24	196
Husband's Income				
Less than $4000	.23	.25	.27	112
$4000–$5999	.05	.05	.13	417
$6000–$7999	− .22	− .23	− .32	395
$8000–$9999	− .05	− .06	− .06	228
$10000–$11999	− .04	− .04	.00	180
$12000 or more	.08	.06	− .08	182
D.K. and N.R.	.07	.07	.00	118
Husband's Occupation				
Upper white collar	.01	.03	.09	616
Lower white collar	− .19	− .20	− .15	284
Blue collar	.06	.05	− .02	732
Wife's Labour Force Status				
Working	− .27	− .27	− .27	585
Not working	.15	.15	.15	1046

(*a*) *Adjusted for marriage duration only.*
(*b*) *Adjusted for age only.*

Appendix C

Analysis of Childspacing Using Life Table Techniques

Analyses of childspacing data collected in fertility surveys have until recently been limited to a study of mean intervals between births and their relationship to various demographic and socio-economic variables. The pitfalls and limitations of using such a measure for an analysis of childspacing from survey data are many. One of the most important and difficult of these problems arises from the fact that the sample is composed of various age cohorts of women many of them having different durations of exposure still left for future fertility in their reproductive period. For any sample of women, past fertility and prospective fertility are a function of her age and marriage duration at the time of the survey. The composite measures constructed from the total sample of women who have been observed for periods of different length are therefore difficult to interpret. For example, the mean family size at the time of the survey is a function of age and marriage duration of women and is not a standardized measure. Similarly, childspacing measures also present problems of interpretation. Period of observation has a direct effect both on closed and open intervals, that is, the interval between successive births and the interval since the most recent birth.

Life-table techniques utilize both closed and open interval distributions to arrive at fertility measures which are adjusted for incomplete periods of observation, that is, not observing a woman for her entire reproductive period. However, even if a woman is observed until the end of the reproductive period, some truncation effect will persist due to the finite nature of the reproductive time period. The effect is not eliminated in the adjusted estimates presented here.[1] All it does is adjust for the unobserved portion of the reproductive period of sample women.

Basic Methodology

Let N^i_x = number of ith closed birth intervals of length x months ($i-1^{th}$ to i^{th} birth)

M^i_x = number of ith open birth intervals of length x months ($i-1^{th}$ to survey date)

B^i_x = number of births in the ith interval

$\sum_{x=0}^{\infty} N^i_x$ = total i^{th} closed intervals

$\sum_{x=0}^{\infty} M^i_x$ = total i^{th} open intervals

$\sum_{x=0}^{\infty} (N^i_x + M^i_x)$ = total sample women who had (i–1) births and open to the risk of ith births

For any particular monthly duration x probability of birth, assuming uniform distribution of events, will be:

$$P^i_x = B^i_x \Big/ \left(\sum_{x=x}^{\infty} N^i_x + M^i_x \right) - \tfrac{1}{2} M^i_x$$

and the probability of non-birth

$$q^i_x = 1 - p^i_x$$

and the cumulative probability of birth delay

$$Q^i_x = \prod_{x=0}^{x} q^i_x$$

[1] Sheps *et al.*, "Truncation Effect in Birth Interval Data."

Table 70 Intervals (Closed and Open) from Marriage to First Birth and Functions Based on Them

	FIRST INTERVAL						
Interval in Months x	*Number of Women at Beginning of Interval* N_x	*Number of Births During the Period* B_x	*Women Lost to Follow Up* M_x	*Adjusted Number of Women Exposed to Childbirth* N^*_x	*Probability of Having a Birth* P_x	*Cumulative Probability of Birth Delay* Q_x	*Standard Error of* Q_x ${}^{S}Q_x$
1–3	1599	20	9	1594.5	.01254	.98746	.0028
4–6	1570	100	23	1558.5	.06416	.92410	.0067
7–9	1447	160	8	1443.0	.11088	.82164	.0097
10–12	1279	192	5	1276.5	.15041	.69806	.0116
13–15	1082	137	13	1075.5	.12738	.60914	.0124
16–18	932	114	15	924.5	.12331	.53402	.0127
19–21	803	90	7	799.5	.11257	.47391	.0127
22–24	706	67	4	704.0	.09517	.42881	.0127
25–27	635	61	2	634.0	.09621	.38755	.0125
28–30	572	48	7	568.5	.08433	.35483	.0123
31–33	517	34	3	515.5	.06596	.33142	.0121
34–36	480	45	2	479.0	.09395	.30029	.0118
37–39	433	36	2	432.0	.09333	.27526	.0116
40–42	395	38	8	391.0	.09719	.24851	.0112
43–45	349	18	4	347.0	.05187	.23562	.0111
46–48	327	32	0	327.0	.09786	.21256	.0107
49–51	295	16	3	293.5	.05451	.20097	.0105

52–54	276	16	2	275.0	.05818	.18928	.0103
55–57	258	12	3	256.5	.04678	.18043	.0101
58–60	243	14	0	243.0	.05761	.17003	.0099
61–63	229	15	3	227.5	.06593	.15882	.0097
64–66	211	6	4	209.0	.02871	.15426	.0096
67–69	201	17	3	199.5	.08521	.14112	.0093
70–72	181	12	1	180.5	.06648	.13173	.0090
73–75	168	14	3	166.5	.08408	.12066	.0088
76–78	151	5	3	149.5	.03344	.11662	.0086
79–81	143	11	3	141.5	.07774	.10755	.0084
82–84	129	6	0	129.0	.04651	.10255	.0082
85–87	123	7	1	122.5	.05714	.09669	.0081
88–90	115	6	1	114.5	.05240	.09162	.0079
91–93	108	1	3	106.5	.00939	.09706	.0084
94–96	104	5	1	103.5	.04831	.08638	.0077
97–108	98	13	4	96.0	.13542	.07468	.0073
109–120	81	9	3	79.5	.11321	.06623	.0070
121–132	69	3	7	65.5	.04580	.06319	.0069
133–144	59	3	5	56.5	.05310	.05984	.0068
145–156	51	5	3	49.5	.10101	.05379	.0066
157–168	43	2	5	40.5	.04938	.05113	.0066
169–180	36	2	5	33.5	.05970	.04808	.0065
181–192	29	0	4	27.0	.00000	.04808	.0065
193–204	25	1	1	24.5	.04082	.04612	.0065
205–336	23	0	23	11.5	.00000	.04612	.0065
337–	0	0	0	0.0	.00000	.04612	.0065

Table 71 Intervals (Closed and Open) between First and Second Birth and Functions Based on Them

	SECOND INTERVAL						
Interval in Months x	*Number of Women at Beginning of Interval* N_x	*Number of Births During the Period* B_x	*Women Lost to Follow Up* M_x	*Adjusted Number of Women Exposed to Childbirth* N^*_x	*Probability of Having a Birth* P_x	*Cumulative Probability of Birth Delay* Q_x	*Standard Error of* Q_x ${}^{s}Q_x$
1–3	1410	0	20	1400.0	.00000	1.00000	.0000
4–6	1390	0	17	1381.5	.00000	1.00000	.0000
7–9	1373	1	15	1365.5	.00243	.99707	.0015
10–12	1354	51	16	1346.0	.03789	.95929	.0054
13–15	1287	106	17	1287.5	.08291	.87976	.0089
16–18	1164	107	12	1158.0	.09240	.79847	.0110
19–21	1045	101	10	1040.0	.09712	.72092	.0123
22–24	934	97	9	929.5	.10436	.64568	.0132
25–27	828	80	12	822.0	.09732	.58285	.0137
28–30	736	74	11	730.5	.10130	.52380	.0139
31–33	651	65	6	648.0	.10031	.47126	.0139
34–36	580	57	9	575.5	.09904	.42459	.0139
37–39	514	48	9	509.5	.09421	.38459	.0137
40–42	457	33	9	452.5	.07293	.35654	.0136
43–45	415	38	5	412.5	.09212	.32370	.0133
46–48	372	29	5	369.5	.07848	.29829	.0131

49–51	338	23	6	335.5	.06866	.27781	.0129
52–54	309	30	2	308.0	.09740	.25075	.0125
55–57	277	22	1	276.5	.07957	.23080	.0122
58–60	254	19	3	252.5	.07525	.21343	.0119
61–63	232	12	1	231.5	.05184	.20237	.0117
64–66	219	14	5	216.5	.06467	.18928	.0114
67–69	200	8	4	198.0	.04040	.18163	.0113
70–72	188	14	1	187.5	.07467	.16807	.0110
73–75	173	8	2	172.0	.04651	.16025	.0108
76–78	163	7	4	161.0	.04348	.15328	.0107
79–81	152	8	5	149.5	.05351	.14508	.0105
82–84	139	4	4	137.0	.02920	.14084	.0104
85–87	131	3	4	129.0	.02236	.13769	.0103
88–90	124	3	3	122.5	.02449	.13432	.0103
91–93	118	5	2	117.0	.04274	.12858	.0101
94–96	111	6	1	110.5	.05430	.12160	.0100
97–108	104	12	7	100.5	.11940	.10708	.0096
109–120	85	5	7	81.5	.06135	.10586	.0100
121–132	73	8	5	70.5	.11348	.09384	.0097
133–144	60	5	4	58.0	.08621	.08576	.0095
145–156	51	1	4	49.0	.02041	.08401	.0095
157–168	46	1	2	47.0	.02222	.08214	.0094
169–180	43	1	11	37.5	.02667	.07995	.0094
181–192	31	1	4	29.0	.03448	.07719	.0095
193–	26	0	26	13.0	.00000		

For any interval i we could construct a table of decrements starting with all sample women with (i-1)th births and indicating decrements for each month x either by births or due to loss to follow up (open interval). Such a table is nothing but a multiple decrement life table and the measures of P^i_x and Q^i_x are analogous to life table functions. Such tables are presented for the first (marriage to first birth) and second birth intervals (tables 70 and 71). Certain interesting patterns are revealed in these tables. First, the probability of giving birth in any month does not reveal any pattern after the first two years, by which time two-thirds of the first births take place. The first year shows increasing probabilities as would be expected since apart from premarital conceptions the first two-thirds of the period are ineligible for legitimate deliveries. The highest probability is reached in the last quarter of the first year, after which probabilities decline throughout the second year, becoming irregular thereafter. After the initial bunching of births the timing is a function of many factors, probably the most important being contraceptive failure which might be expected to be distributed randomly. Two factors ignored here are the effect of a reduction in fecundity by age and mortality.

Comparison with first interval reveals that second births are delayed longer than first births, in part because of the inclusion of illegitimate conceptions in the first interval. The highest probabilities are reached between 21 months and 36 months. Cumulative probability of having a birth reaches .5 only after 30 months and .75 after 54 months, much longer than in the case of first birth.

Parity Progression Ratios

Parity progression ratios can be calculated for any marriage cohort by following them for their reproductive period. This is not possible in a cross-section sample as the women are at various stages of their reproductive career. Using life-table techniques as outlined in the earlier section we can compute parity progression ratios which are derived from the observed portions of the entire sample. It will be seen that the probability of birth becomes zero after a fairly long duration, and cumulative birth delay reaches a constant value. If we define i^{th} Parity Progression Ratio (PPR) as the proportion of women who pass from (i-1th) to i^{th} parity, it is given by $1\text{-}Q^i_{k+1}$, where K is the last interval where there is a non-zero birth probability.

Life-Table Mean Interval

For any i, a life-table mean interval can be calculated by the formula:

$$\overline{X}^{i} = \sum_{x=o}^{k} \frac{x\,(Q_x^i - Q_{x+1}^i)}{1 - Q_{k+1}^i}$$

These values are presented in table 29 of chapter 3.

Appendix D

Table 72 Base Populations for Percentages Portrayed in Figures 5–6

	ROMAN CATHOLIC WOMEN				PROTESTANT WOMEN			
	Less than Grade 12		*Grade 12 or Above*		*Less than Grade 12*		*Grade 12 or Above*	
	Foreign Born	*Native Born*	*Foreign Born*	*Native Born*	*Foreign Born*	*Native Born*	*Foreign Born*	*Native Born*
1963								
January			166	97	90	210	109	263
April			169	97	91	213	109	267
July			170	98	93	219	111	273
October			172	99	94	225	114	277
1964								
January			173	100	94	227	115	278
April			174	100	94	229	116	278
July			175	100	95	232	116	282
October			176	101	96	240	117	284

1965								
January			179	102	96	242	117	285
April			181	102	97	243	117	287
July	57	44	183	105	99	247	120	289
October	59	46	186	106	101	252	120	292
1966								
January	59	47	187	107	101	252	121	294
April	59	47	190	107	104	252	121	298
July	59	48	192	109	108	258	121	304
October	61	51	195	110	110	265	125	306
1967								
January	61	51	195	111	111	266	126	307
April	61	52	195	112	112	270	126	308
July	61	55	196	114	114	278	127	313
October	64	56	196	115	117	284	128	319

Appendix E

Analysis of Oral Contraceptive Use through Multiple Decrement Life Table Techniques

Actuarial approaches to the measurement of contraceptive effectiveness are of recent origin. Multiple decrement life tables, long established in actuarial work, have recently been adopted to the study of attrition in the use of particular contraceptive methods and in comparing the effectiveness of oral contraception in different populations.[1] The life-table approach not only provides a way of constructing duration-specific termination rates but also makes it possible to include in the construction of rates both the continuing users as well as those who have stopped contraceptive use.

Termination by Cause

The distribution of the first segments of use of the 732 women who started using the pill on or after January 1962 by length and termination status is presented in table 73. A serious limitation of the data for analysis is sample size. Even after grouping in three monthly intervals, the numbers are too small in many categories to insure

[1] Potter, "The Multiple Decrement Life Table as an Approach to the Measurement of Use Effectiveness and Demographic Effectiveness of Contraception," Freedman and Takeshita, *Family Planning in Taiwan.* Jones and Mauldin, "Use of Oral Contraceptives: With Special Reference to Developing Countries."

stability. The emphasis therefore will be on general pattern rather than on specific rates. A much larger sample would be necessary to validate decrement rates for small durations. Standard Errors are presented, computed by techniques suggested by Potter and others.[2]

The following notation is used:

x = denotes durations in three monthly units

$N_x^{(T)}$ = number of women using the pill at the beginning of the quarter

P_x = number of women terminating use of pill to become pregnant in quarter x

M_x = number of women terminating use of pill for medical and health reasons during the quarter x

O_x = number of women terminating use of pill for all other reasons during the quarter x

T_x = $P_x + M_x + O_x$

W_x = number of users last observed during quarter x.

The decrement rates for various causes by length of first segment are presented in table 74. These rates have been called net rates to distinguish them from the absolute rates calculated later in this section. The net rates are calculated by the formulae

$$q_x^{(p)} = P_x/N_x^{*\,(T)} \text{ etc.}$$

where

$$N_x^{*(T)} = N_x^{(T)} - (W_x/2)$$

to make allowance for the fact that if the loss rate is uniform, those who stop use in a given quarter are on an average exposed only half the time to the risk of pregnancy or other decrements.

$$q_x^{(T)} = q_x^{(p)} + q_x^{(m)} + q_x^{(0)}$$

and

$$p_x^{(T)} = 1 - q_x^{(T)}$$

and

$$P_x^{(T)} = \prod_{x=1}^{x} p_x^{(T)}$$

$P_x^{(T)}$ is the familiar continuation rate at the end of x quarters of use.

[2] Freedman and Takeshita, *Family Planning in Taiwan,* Appendix X-2, pp. 469-70.

Table 73 First Segments of Oral Contraceptive Use * by Length of Use and Termination Status (1 January 1962 to November 1967)

Months of Exposure	TERMINATION *Planning Pregnancy*	*Medical, Health*	*Others*	*Total*	*Continuing Users*	*All Segments*
x	P_x	M_x	O_x	T_x	W_x	$T_x + W_x$
1–3	15	64	30	109	32	141
4–6	10	33	12	55	31	86
7–9	12	19	13	44	24	68
10–12	6	8	17	31	24	55
13–15	7	15	4	26	27	53
16–18	3	4	4	11	19	30
19–21	2	3	3	8	26	34
22–24	2	9	3	14	23	37
25–27	6	7	2	15	29	44
28–30	2	1	5	8	13	21
31–33	3	5	3	11	21	32
34–36	2	1	2	5	19	24
37–39	2	1	1	4	16	20
40–42	3	2	5	10	9	19
43–45	2	2	1	5	10	15
46–48	1	0	0	1	13	14
49 or more	2	1	0	3	36	39
Total	80	175	105	360	372	732

**First segment refers to the period of use from the time the method was first used to either termination or to the time of the survey. Loss to follow up, a third type of decrement which must be dealt with in analysing registration statistics, is logically excluded as a possibility in survey data.*

Absolute Rates of Decrement

The problems of interpreting net decrement rates, where the decrements are made up of competing risks, are well recognized in multiple decrement theory.[3] The stated net rates are not independent of each other. For comparative purposes it is probably more meaningful to look at the underlying absolute or true rates of decrement for each type of determination. (In the terminology of Potter and Tietze, these absolute or true rates are gross rates and the earlier rates are net rates.) These rates called "gross rates" by Tietze and Potter are the rates that would be observed if other competing risks were not present. The formulae for constructing these are:

$$q_x'^{(p)} = P_x/N_x^{**(p)}$$

where

$$N_x^{**(P)} = N_x^{(T)} - \tfrac{1}{2}(M_x + O_x + W_x)$$

and similar expressions for q_x' (m) and q_x' (o).

The relationship between the net and absolute rate can be expressed as:

$$q_x'^{(p)} = \frac{q_x^{(p)}}{1 - \frac{1}{2}(q_x^{(m)} + q_x^{(o)})}$$

or in general

$$= \frac{q_x^{(p)}}{1 - \frac{1}{2}(\Sigma q_x^{(i)} - q_x^{(p)})}$$

and similar expressions for $q_x'^{(m)}$ and $q_x'^{(o)}$.

These absolute rates along with the corresponding continuation rates and standard errors are presented in table 75. The patterns of discontinuation are virtually identical with those in table 74.

Relationship between Single Decrement and Total Decrement Continuation Rates

As the single most commonly used measure in effectiveness studies is the continuation rate after specific durations, it will be of interest to look at the relationship between total continuation rates and the decomposed single decrement continuation rates. The merit of

[3] Jordan, *Life Contingencies.*

absolute rates of decrement is that, apart from giving true independent measures of decrement, the products of the single decrement continuation rates are found to be very close to the total continuation rates when the values of the q's are small, which is often the case in effectiveness studies. Table 76 shows the products of the absolute continuation rates by cause along with the total continuation rates reported earlier in table 74. The differences are very small and often no greater than rounding errors. Algebraically it can be shown that the differences consist of terms which are third or higher powers of q.

(The product of the absolute continuation rates for a time period is:

$$\prod_i 1 - \frac{q_i}{1 - \frac{\Sigma q - q_i}{2}}$$

$$= \prod_i \left[1 - q_i \left\{ 1 + \left(\frac{\Sigma q - q_i}{2} \right) \right. \right.$$

$$\left. \left. + \left(\frac{\Sigma q - q_i}{2}^2 \right) + \ldots \right\} \right]$$

$$= \prod_i \left[1 - q_i - q_i \frac{\Sigma q}{2} \right.$$

$$\left. + \frac{q_i^2}{2} + O(q^3) + O(q^4) \ldots \right]$$

$$= 1 - \Sigma q - \frac{(\Sigma q)^2}{2} + \frac{\Sigma q^2}{2}$$

$$+ \sum_{i \neq j} q_i q_j + O(q^3) + O(q^4) \ldots$$

$$= 1 - \Sigma q + O(q^3) + O(q^4) \ldots$$

$$\doteqdot 1 - \Sigma q \text{ when q's are small}$$

$$\doteqdot \text{total continuation rate.)}$$

Only for values of q as large as .2 does the difference become significant. In the continuous case of course, the product will be exactly equal to the total continuation rate.

Table 74 Decrement Rates by Cause of Termination and Length of Exposure

Months of Exposure	Number at Beginning	Adjusted Number Exposed	PROBABILITY OF TERMINATION (*Net Rates*) Planning Pregnancy	Medical, Health	Others	Total	Cumulative Continuation Rate	Standard Error of Cumulative Rate
x	$N_x^{(T)}$	$N_x^{*(T)}$	$q_x^{(p)}$	$q_x^{(m)}$	$q_x^{(o)}$	$q_x^{(T)}$	$P_x^{(T)}$	S.E.*
1–3	732	716	.0209	.0894	.0419	.1522	.8478	.013
4–6	591	576	.0174	.0573	.0208	.0955	.7668	.016
7–9	505	493	.0243	.0385	.0264	.0892	.6984	.017
10–12	437	425	.0141	.0188	.0400	.0729	.6475	.019
13–15	382	369	.0190	.0407	.0108	.0705	.6019	.019
16–18	329	319	.0094	.0125	.0125	.0344	.5811	.020
19–21	299	286	.0070	.0105	.0105	.0280	.5648	.020
22–24	265	253	.0079	.0356	.0119	.0554	.5336	.020
25–27	228	213	.0282	.0329	.0094	.0705	.4960	.021
28–30	184	178	.0112	.0056	.0281	.0449	.4738	.022
31–33	163	153	.0196	.0327	.0196	.0719	.4397	.022
34–36	131	122	.0164	.0082	.0164	.0410	.4217	.023
37–39	107	99	.0202	.0101	.0101	.0404	.4046	.023
40–42	87	83	.0361	.0241	.0602	.1204	.3559	.025
43–45	68	63	.0317	.0317	.0159	.0793	.3276	.026
46–48	53	47	.0213	.0000	.0000	.0213	.3206	.027
49+	39							

*– S.E. of $P_x^{(T)} = P_x^{(T)} \sum_{x=1}^{X} \frac{q_x^{(T)}}{p_x^{(T)} N_x^{*(T)}}$ ½

Simpler formulae for the calculation of approximate standard errors have been suggested by Tietze: for discussion of the relative merits of different formulae, see Freedman and Takeshita, 1969, Appendix X-2.

Table 75 Absolute Decrement Rates and Continuation Rates by Cause and Length of Exposure

	PLANNING PREGNANCY			MEDICAL AND HEALTH			OTHERS		
Months of Exposure	*Decrement Rate*	*Continuation Rate*	*S.E. of Continuation Rate*	*Decrement Rate*	*Continuation Rate*	*S.E. of Continuation Rate*	*Decrement Rate*	*Continuation Rate*	*S.E. of Continuation Rate*
x	$q_x'^{(p)}$	$p_x'^{(p)}$		$q_x'^{(m)}$	$p_x'^{(m)}$		$q_x'^{(o)}$	$p_x'^{(o)}$	
1–3	.0224	.9776	.005	.0923	.9077	.011	.0443	.9557	.008
4–6	.0181	.9599	.008	.0584	.8547	.013	.0216	.9350	.010
7–9	.0251	.9358	.010	.0395	.8209	.015	.0273	.9095	.012
10–12	.0145	.9222	.012	.0193	.8051	.016	.0407	.8725	.014
13–15	.0195	.9042	.013	.0413	.7718	.017	.0111	.8628	.015
16–18	.0095	.8956	.014	.0126	.7620	.018	.0126	.8519	.016
19–21	.0071	.8893	.015	.0106	.7540	.018	.0106	.8429	.016
22–24	.0081	.8820	.015	.0360	.7269	.020	.0122	.8326	.017
25–27	.0288	.8567	.018	.0335	.7025	.021	.0097	.8246	.018
28–30	.0114	.8469	.019	.0057	.6985	.021	.0283	.8012	.020
31–33	.0201	.8299	.021	.0334	.6752	.023	.0201	.7851	.022
34–36	.0166	.8161	.023	.0083	.6695	.024	.0166	.7720	.023
37–39	.0204	.7995	.025	.0103	.6627	.024	.0103	.7641	.025
40–42	.0377	.7693	.030	.0253	.6459	.026	.0621	.7167	.031
43–45	.0325	.7443	.034	.0325	.6249	.029	.0164	.7040	.033
46–48	.0213	.7285	.036	.0000	.6249	.029	.0000	.7049	.033
49+									

Table 76 Comparison of Absolute Continuation Rates by Cause and Total Continuation Rate

	CONTINUATION RATES					
Months	*Planning Pregnancy*	*Medical, Health*	*Others*	*Product of Columns* (2) × (3) × (4)	*Total Continuation Rate*	*Column* (5) *Minus Column* (6)[a]
1–3	.9776	.9077	.9557	.8480	.8478	.0002
4–6	.9599	.8547	.9350	.7671	.7668	.0003
7–9	.9358	.8209	.9095	.6987	.6984	.0003
10–12	.9222	.8051	.8725	.6478	.6475	.0003
13–15	.9042	.7718	.8628	.6022	.6019	.0003
16–18	.8956	.7620	.8519	.5814	.5812	.0002
19–21	.8893	.7540	.8429	.5652	.5649	.0003
22–24	.8820	.7269	.8326	.5339	.5336	.0003
25–27	.8567	.7025	.8246	.4962	.4960	.0002
28–30	.8469	.6985	.8012	.4740	.4737	.0003
31–33	.8299	.6752	.7851	.4399	.4396	.0003
34–36	.8161	.6695	.7720	.4219	.4216	.0003
37–39	.7995	.6627	.7641	.4048	.4046	.0002
40–42	.7693	.6459	.7167	.3561	.3559	.0002
43–45	.7443	.6249	.7049	.3279	.3277	.0002
46–48	.7285	.6249	.7049	.3209	.3207	.0002
49+						

[a] *Column (5) will always be greater than Column (6) because of approximate formulae used for the discrete cases. However, the differences are not cumulative and hence need not increase with duration. In the continuous case, the two columns will of course be exactly equal.*

Appendix F

Multiple Classification Analysis of Attitudes towards Abortion

As many fertility and socio-economic variables are interrelated, it is difficult to assess the relative importance of these without appropriate multivariate analysis. Two statistical measures for each category of each independent variable are shown in table 77. "Unadjusted" deviations are the deviations of category "mean abortion index" from "mean abortion index for all women." "Adjusted" deviations are these category-specific deviations after the effects of other independant variables are taken into account.

Religion seems to be the most powerful predictor. After adjusting for religiosity and for all the other eight predictors there is still a difference of 1.3 in the abortion index of Catholics and non-Catholics. Religiosity as measured by church attendance is also important. After controlling for the other independent variables, a difference of 1.7 remains between the abortion index of those who don't attend church and those who attend most often. The positive relation between education and attitudes towards abortion persists after controlling for other predictors, but there is very little difference between the educational categories, after nine years of schooling. The association of size of birthplace and abortion attitude is also diminished when control is imposed for other factors. The relationship of husband's income to abortion attitude is diminished but remains strong after control for the other predictors.

For age and desired family size, the adjusted deviations are lower in magnitude than unadjusted deviations, but the patterns are essentially the same and the differences substantial in the case of desired family size. Why younger women are less liberal than older women is a somewhat perplexing question and requires further investigation. It may be associated with the previously observed tendency for those who have experienced a contraceptive failure to be more liberal in their attitudes towards abortion. Age and the risk of unwanted pregnancy are positively associated.

When controlled for other predictors, the relationship of current contraceptive use to attitudes towards abortion loses much of its significance. Only women using mechanical methods of condom and diaphragm or rhythm vary from the overall norm. Women who had an unwanted pregnancy in terms of number still seem to be slightly more liberal than other women even after taking account of other factors.

The combined effects of the predictors on the attitudes towards abortion are presented in table 78. The three situational variables—desired family size, current contraceptive method, and planning status of last pregnancy explain only ten per cent of the variance in the abortion attitude scores. When only religion and religiosity are used as predictors the variance explained is 23 per cent. When as many as nine predictors are used, 31 per cent of the variation is explained.[1] In spite of using as many as nine independent variables, the fact that we are able to explain only about one-third of the variance in abortion attitude scores suggests the complex nature of attitudes on a sensitive issue such as abortion.

[1] Westoff, Moore, and Ryder, "Structure of Attitudes Towards Abortion," p. 27. The proportion of variance explained in our sample is considerably higher than the 21 per cent explained in the U.S. sample by Westoff and Ryder. See their article, "Structure of Attitudes Towards Abortion."

Table 77 Multiple Classification Analysis of Abortion Attitude Scores in Relation to Selected Demographic and Socio-Economic Characteristics

Predictors	*Unadjusted Deviations from the Grand Mean*	*Deviations Adjusted for Religion and Religiosity*	*Deviations Adjusted for All Other Predictors*	*Number of Women*
Religion				
Catholic	−1.73	−1.44 (a)	−.95	414
Non-Catholic	.75	.62 (a)	.39	1005
Religiosity				
Don't attend	.99	.63 (b)	.66	476
Rarely attend	.19	.08 (b)	.17	422
Less than 5 times a month	−.88	−.48 (b)	−.61	351
5 or more times a month	−1.47	−1.01 (b)	−1.02	170
Education				
8 years or less of schooling	−1.27	−.68	−.35	289
9–11 years of schooling	.25	.14	.02	545
12 years	.39	.23	.18	356
Some university	.80	.41	.16	229
Husband's Income				
Less than $5,000	−1.59	−1.03	−.58	205
$5,000–$5,999	−.33	−.20	−.40	257
$6,000–$7,999	−.05	−.08	−.10	385
$8,000–$9,999	.58	.33	.29	221
$10,000 or more	1.05	.68	.50	351
Size of Birthplace				
Less than 5,000	−.74	−.46	−.33	329
5,000–49,999	−.46	−.14	−.07	347

50,000–499,999	.24	.06	.02	200
500,000 or more	.68	.27	.16	535
Age				
18–24	−.65	−.68	−.51	140
25–29	−.25	−.35	−.34	289
30–34	.14	.19	.12	278
35–39	.24	.26	.20	324
40 or above	.16	.16	.22	388
Desired Family Size				
0 or 1	.95	.40	.78	32
2	.34	.08	.14	473
3	.15	.16	.17	436
4	−.31	−.07	−.24	380
5	−1.23	−.65	−.45	39
6 or more	−1.56	−1.08	−.93	59
Current Method of Contraception				
Mechanical (condom and diaphragm)	.81	.57	.30	267
Oral pills and IUD	.34	.14	.08	470
Chemical and others	−.22	.01	.08	114
Rhythm	−1.65	−.56	−.75	81
None, at risk	−.69	−.44	−.16	265
None, not at risk	−.17	−.14	−.11	222
Last Pregnancy Status				
Number failure	.51	.32	.36	204
Spacing failure	−.09	−.07	.05	195
All others	−.08	−.05	−.02	1020

(a) Controlled for religiosity only.
(b) Controlled for religion only.
Unadjusted deviations may vary slightly from figures in tables in chapter 6 because fewer cases were used in MCA.

Table 78 Partial Beta Co-Efficients of Predictors and Variance Explained on Abortion Index *

	Partial Beta Co-Efficients		
Predictors	*Three Predictors*	*Two Predictors*	*Nine Predictors*
Religion		.367	.241
Religiosity		−.218	−.243
Education			.081
Husband's Income			.176
Size of Birthplace			.067
Age of Wife			.123
Desired Family Size	−.138		−.116
Current Method of Contraception	.235		.096
Last Pregnancy Status	.085		.062
Multiple Correlation Co-Efficient	.317	.484	.553
Variance Explained	10%	23%	31%

**The Beta co-efficients presented here are derived from the multiple classification analysis. These indicate the relative importance of the various predictors in their joint explanation of the dependent variable. However, they are only moderately good substitutes for the partial correlation co-efficients. For a technical discussion of the MCA, see Frank Andrews, James Morgan, and John Sonquist,* Multiple Classification Analysis, *Institute for Social Research, University of Michigan, November 1969.*

Bibliography

Allingham, J. D.; Balakrishnan, T. R.; and Kantner, J. F. "Time Series of Growth in Use of Oral Contraceptives and the Differential Diffusion of Oral Anovulants." *Population Studies* 23, no. 1 (1969): 43–51.

Allingham, J. D.; Balakrishnan, T. R.; and Kantner, J. F. "The End of Rapid Increase in the Use of Oral Anovulants? Some Problems in the Interpretation of Time Series of Oral Use Among Married Women." *Demography*, 7 (1970): 31–41.

Andrews, Frank; Morgan, James; and Sonquist, John. *Multiple Classification Analysis.* Institute for Social Research, University of Michigan. November, 1969.

Balakrishnan, T. R.; Allingham, J. D.; and Kantner, J. F. "Analysis of Oral Contraceptive Use Through Multiple Decrement Life Table Techniques." *Demography*, 7 (1970): 459–65.

Balakrishnan, T. R.; Shan, Ross; Allingham, J. D.; and Kantner, J. F. "Attitudes Towards Abortion of Married Women in Metropolitan Toronto." *Social Biology*, 19 (1972): 35–42.

Becker, G. S. "An Economic Analysis of Fertility" in *Demographic and Economic Change in Developed Countries.* National Bureau of Economic Research. 1960.

Blake, Judith. "Americanization of Catholic Reproductive Ideals." *Population Studies*, 20 (1966): 20–43.

Blake, Judith. "Are Babies Consumer Durables?" *Population Studies*, 22 (1968): 5–25.

Bogue, Donald. *Principles of Demography*. New York: John Wiley and Sons. 1969.

Boyce, R. M.; and Osborn, R. W. "Therapeutic Abortion in a Canadian City." *Canadian Medical Association Journal*, 103 (1970): 310–27.

British Medical Journal. "Oral Contraception and Thromboembolism." *British Medical Journal*, 2 (1968): 187.

Chaudhury, Rafiqul Huda. "Relative Income and Fertility." Ph.D. dissertation. Johns Hopkins University, 1973.

Chen, F. L.; Chang, M. C.; Sun, T. H.; and Gernada, George P. "First Island Wide Pill Acceptor Follow-up Survey, 1968." Interim Report of Survey of Research Projects. Taiwan Provincial Institute of Family Planning (preliminary). 1969.

Chiang, C. L. *Introduction to Stochastic Processes in Biostatistics*. New York: Wiley and Company. 1969.

Coombs, Lolagene; Freedman, Ronald; Freedman, Judith; and Pratt, William. "Premarital Pregnancy and Labor Force Status Before and After Marriage." *American Journal of Sociology*, 75 (1970): 800–820.

Destler, Harriet P. "Work Before the First Birth: Its Relation to Fertility and Contraceptive Practice." Master's thesis. Johns Hopkins University. 1972.

Dominion Bureau of Statistics. *Census of Canada, 1961*. Bulletin 4–1–7.

Easterlin, Richard. "Toward a Socio-Economic Theory of Fertility." Pp. 127–56 in Freedman, *et al.* (eds.), *Fertility and Family Planning*. 1969.

Freedman, *et al. Family Planning, Sterility and Population Growth*. McGraw-Hill. 1959.

Freedman, Ronald; and Bumpass, Larry. "Fertility Expectations in the U.S.: 1962–1964." *Population Index*, 32 (1966): 181–97.

Freedman, Ronald; and Coombs, Lolagene. "Childspacing and Family Economic Position." *American Sociological Review*, 31 (1966): 631–48.

Freedman, Ronald; and Takeshita, John Y. *Family Planning in Taiwan*. Princeton, New Jersey: Princeton University Press. 1969.

Goldberg, David; Sharp, Harry; and Freedman, Ronald. "The Stability and Reliability of Expected Family Size Data." *Milbank Memorial Fund Quarterly*, 37, no. 4 (1959): 369–85.

Government of Canada. *Report of the Royal Commission on The Status of Women in Canada.* 1970.

Griffith, Janet. "Family Size Norms and Informal Social Control." Ph.D. dissertation. Johns Hopkins University. 1973.

Henripin, Jacques. *Trends and Factors of Fertility in Canada.* Statistics Canada. 1972.

Henripin, Jacques; and Legare, J. "Recent Trends in Canadian Fertility." *The Canadian Review of Sociology and Anthropology,* 8 (1971): 106–18.

Jones, Elise F.; and Westoff, Charles F. "Attitudes Toward Abortion in the United States in 1970 and the Trend Since 1965." Research paper prepared for the Commission on Population Growth and the American Future. 1972.

Jones, Gavin; and Mauldin, Parker. "Use of Oral Contraceptives: With Special Reference to Developing Countries." *Studies in Family Planning* no. 24 (1967): 1–13.

Jordan, C. W. *Life Contingencies.* The Society of Actuaries. 1952.

Kantner, J. F.; Allingham, J. D.; and Balakrishnan, T. R. "Oral Contraception and the Fertility Decline in Canada, 1958–1968. A First Look at a Crucial Component in the Argument." Paper presented to Population Association of America. Boston. 17 April 1968.

Kantner, J. F.; and Allingham, J. D. "American Attitudes on Population Policy: Recent Trends." *Studies in Family Planning,* 30 (1968): 1–7.

Krotki, Karol; and Lapierre, Evelyne. "La fécondité au Canada selon la religion, l'origine ethnique et l'étât matrimonial." *Population,* 23, no. 5 (1968): 815–34.

Lavis, Donald. "Ontario: The Pill and the Birth Rate 1960–1967." Master's thesis. University of Western Ontario. 1970.

Lorimer, Frank. *Culture and Human Fertility.* UNESCO. 1954.

Namboodiri, N. Krishnan. "Some Observations on the Economic Framework for Fertility Analysis." *Population Studies,* 26 (1972): 185–206.

Parakulam, George. "Wives Who Have Unwanted Children." Master's thesis. University of Western Ontario. 1970.

Potter, R. G. "Some Physical Correlates of Fertility Control in the United States." *Proceedings of the International Population Conference. New York,* 1 (1961): 106–16.

Potter, R. G. "Birth Intervals: Structure and Change." *Population Studies*, 17 (1963): 155–66.

Potter, R. G. "Application of Life Table Techniques to Measurement of Contraceptive Effectiveness." *Demography*, 3, no. 2 (1966): 297–304.

Potter, R. G. "The Multiple Decrement Life Table as an Approach to the Measurement of Use Effectiveness and Demographic Effectiveness of Contraception." Pp. 869–83 in *Contributed Papers: Sydney Conference of the International Union for the Scientific Study of Population.* 1967.

Presser, Harriet. "The Timing of First Birth, Female Roles and Black Fertility." Paper read at the 1970 Annual Meetings of the Population Association of America. Atlanta, Georgia. 1970.

Rossi, A. S. "Public Views on Abortion." Pp. 26–53 in Guttmacher, A. F., ed., *The Case for Legalized Abortion Now*. Berkeley: California Diablo Press. 1967.

Ryder, N. B.; and Westoff, C. F. "Use of Oral Contraception in the United States, 1965." *Science* 153 (3741). (1966): 1199–1205.

Ryder, Norman; and Westoff, Charles. "The Trend of Expected Parity in the U.S., 1955, 1960 and 1965." *Population Index*, 33, no. 2 (1967): 153–67.

Ryder, N. B.; and Westoff, C. F. "The United States: The Pill and the Birth Rate: 1960–1965." *Studies in Family Planning*, no. 20 (1967): 1–3.

Ryder, Norman. "Comments." Pp. S65–S69 in *New Economic Approaches to Fertility. Journal of Political Economy* 81, no. 2 (1973).

Ryder, Norman; and Westoff, Charles. "Wanted and Unwanted Fertility in the United States: 1965 and 1970." Commission on Population Growth and the American Future. *Research Reports.* Volume 1, *Demographic and Social Aspects of Population Growth.* 1973.

Ryder, Norman; and Westoff, Charles. *Reproduction in the United States 1965*. Princeton University Press. 1971.

Sheps, M. C., *et al.* "Birth Intervals: Artifact and Reality." *Contributed Papers, Sydney Conference of The International Union for the Scientific Study of Population.* 1967.

Sheps, M. C., *et al.* "Truncation Effects in Birth Interval Data." *Journal of the American Statistical Association*, 65 (1970): 678–93.

Srinivasan, K. "Findings and Implications of a Correlation Analysis of the Closed and Open Birth Intervals." *Demography*, 7, no. 4 (1970): 401–10.

Statistics Canada. *Vital Statistics of Canada Annual Reports.* 1969.

Tietze, C. "Probability of Pregnancy Resulting from a Single Unprotected Coitus." *Fertility and Sterility*, 11, no. 5 (1961): 485–88.

U.S. Department of Commerce. *Birth Expectations and Fertility, June 1972.* Current Population Reports, Series P-20, no. 248. 1973.

Veevers, Jean. "The Liberalization of the Canadian Abortion Laws." Pp. 33–39 in Boydell, *et al.* (eds.), *Critical Issues in Canadian Society.* Toronto: Holt, Rinehart and Winston of Canada, Ltd. 1971.

Westoff, C. E.; and Ryder, N. B. "Duration of Use of Oral Contraception in the U.S., 1960–1965." *U.S. Public Health Reports*, 84, no. 4 (1968): 277–87.

Westoff, C. E.; Moore, E. C.; and Ryder, N. B. "The Structure of Attitudes Towards Abortion." *Milbank Memorial Fund Quarterly*, 47 (1969): 11–37.

Westoff, C. E., ed. *Toward the End of Growth: Population in America.* New Jersey: Prentice-Hall, 1973.

Whelpton, Pascal; Campbell, Arthur; and Patterson, John. *Fertility and Family Planning in the U.S.* Princeton, New Jersey: Princeton University Press. 1966.

Zelnik, Melvin; and Kantner, John. "Sexuality, Contraception, and Pregnancy Among Pre-adult Females in the United States." Commission on Population Growth and the American Future. *Research Reports*, Volume 1, *Demographic and Social Aspects of Population Growth.* Westoff, Charles; and Parke, Robert Jr. (eds.). 1973.

Index